Coping with PMS

...rah Ahmed is a specialty registrar in the general practice department of a ...ndon hospital. Following her training at Cardiff University, she developed ... interest in women's health while working as a house officer in obstetrics ...d gynaecology in the Birmingham area. She went on to work in the ...omen's Health Department at Queen's Hospital, Romford, and at King ...eorge Hospital, Ilford. An associate member of the Medical Journalists' ...sociation, Farah has been published in several women's lifestyle maga-...es, including *Good Housekeeping* and *Vogue* (India), and has appeared ... television to provide health advice. She is currently a medical reviewer ... popular health website *WebMD*. Her long-term goal is to become a GP ...pecializing in women's health.

...mma Cordle is a senior house officer working in the east London area. She ... currently in a specialist training post in obstetrics and gynaecology. After ...mpleting her training at Leicester Warwick University Medical School, ...mma spent time in hospitals around the Leicester area and in Ipswich, ...here she developed an interest in women's health. From 2005 to 2006, ...e spent a year doing research in obstetrics at Leicester Royal Infirmary, ...r which she was awarded a first-class honours degree. She has worked ... the Women's Health Department at Queen's Hospital, Romford, and at ...ng George Hospital, Ilford. Her long-term goal is to become a hospital ...nsultant in obstetrics and gynaecology.

Overcoming Common Problems Series

Selected titles

A full list of titles is available from Sheldon Press,
36 Causton Street, London SW1P 4ST and on our website at
www.sheldonpress.co.uk

Overcoming Common Problems

Coping with PMS

DR FARAH AHMED
and
DR EMMA CORDLE

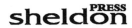
sheldon**PRESS**

First published in Great Britain in 2009

Sheldon Press
36 Causton Street
London SW1P 4ST

British Library Cataloguing-in-Publication Data
A catalogue record for this book is available from the British Library

ISBN 978–1–84709–063–8

1 3 5 7 9 10 8 6 4 2

Typeset by Fakenham Photosetting Ltd, Fakenham, Norfolk
Printed in Great Britain by Ashford Colour Press

Produced on paper from sustainable forests

I dedicate this book to my beloved parents, Shamim and Zia, without whom I would be nothing; to my beautiful sister, Amber, for always being there for me; and, finally, to my darling husband Imran for being the wind beneath my wings.

Farah Ahmed

First and foremost, I give thanks to God for his help with writing this book, which I hope will be a great help to many women.

I would like to dedicate it to my sister, Susie, and my mum, Heather. Thanks so much for your help and patience: you are an inspiration and I love you both with all my heart.

Emma Cordle

Contents

Note to the reader

This is not a medical book and is not intended to replace advice from your doctor. Consult your pharmacist or doctor if you believe you have any of the symptoms described, and if you think you might need medical help.

Foreword

Severe premenstrual syndrome (PMS) continues to be poorly understood and, in many cases, inadequately managed for a number of reasons: failure to train professionals to manage the condition, either at undergraduate or postgraduate level; societal prejudices; and ignorance. It is often very difficult for a woman with severe PMS to have her symptoms taken seriously either by her partner or the medical profession. The media still continue to pose the question: 'Is it PMS or are you just a grumpy woman?' The problem is that the majority of women will experience minor physical and emotional changes premenstrually. However, when severe (in approximately 5 per cent of cases), these symptoms can lead to a breakdown in interpersonal relationships and interfere with normal activities. PMS can be the cause of considerable ill-health and, at times, even death.

I believe this handbook will be an invaluable guide to women who have PMS. It will help them – and their partners – to understand what causes the symptoms, and how these symptoms can affect their quality of life and personal and professional relationships. The book cuts through the mythology that, for example, 'evening primrose oil is the universal panacea'. By the time they get to health professionals, women with severe PMS have already optimized their eating habits, changed their lifestyles and tried many of the over-the-counter remedies, often with little or no benefit. This handbook will guide those who have PMS through the many treatments available, clarifying what the true, evidence-based management options are. Armed with this information, women will be able to make a truly informed choice about which treatments will suit their individual needs. And to ensure that this informative text is in touch with those needs, Farah Ahmed and Emma Cordle liaised closely with the National Association for Premenstrual Syndrome (NAPS; www.pms.org.uk), the PMS patient advocacy society.

Coping with PMS will empower women with the condition to seek appropriate help from their primary care physicians and to request referrals if they need more help from hospital specialists.

Nick Panay, Consultant Gynaecologist
Queen Charlotte's and Chelsea Hospital, London, and
Chairman of the National Association for Premenstrual Syndrome

1

Introduction

As doctors, and women, we are constantly approached by friends, family and just about anyone wanting to know the truth about pre-menstrual syndrome (PMS). We've both had first-hand experience with PMS and are fed up with constantly hearing that it doesn't exist. How on earth can the 80 per cent of all women who are affected by PMS be wrong and accept that it's simply all made up?

There are so many conflicting opinions on the causes, and even the sheer existence of PMS has been called into question. We took it upon ourselves to get to the bottom of this mystery condition and try to set the record straight once and for all.

Thankfully, PMS is now recognized as a genuine condition by the Royal College of Obstetricians and Gynaecologists, who have waded through all the misinformation to give clear guidance to doctors on what treatments are useful and for which woman.

PMS is the name given to a wide range of symptoms which occur in the days before a period, affecting up to 80 per cent of women to some degree. Symptoms may be physical, emotional or psychological. Some women are able to accept these symptoms as an unpleasant but unavoidable part of life. They may take some painkillers and require a bit more TLC than usual, but on the whole they are able to get on with their lives in spite of it.

However, a significant number of women find that PMS has a major effect on their enjoyment of life, their relationships, jobs and home life, and even their ability to function on almost any level, in the time just before and during their period. Around 5 to 10 per cent of women suffer with severe PMS. This may involve depression, tearfulness, terrible anxiety, or physical symptoms such as cramps, headaches or breast tenderness which are severe enough to stop them getting on with their lives.

Certain women have been shown to be at higher risk of PMS: in particular, those who smoke, are overweight or have a family history of it. Nevertheless, many women who don't have any of these risk factors still suffer, and want to know what they can do to help themselves.

For many years women have been fobbed off, ignored or just told to pull themselves together, but it's not always quite that simple. Despite being formally acknowledged for over 50 years, PMS is still not widely understood or recognized by many in today's society, even by some in the medical profession, although this is finally beginning to change. There is a huge range of remedies for PMS, both medical and alternative; knowing what's effective and what's not can seem an impossible mystery, or a kind of lottery.

In December 2007 the Royal College of Obstetricians and Gynaecologists – the leading medical professional organization for women's healthcare in the UK – published guidelines for doctors and health professionals on the best management of women with PMS. These guidelines show that at last PMS is being recognized, and the myths and mysteries around its treatment are being properly investigated, with good evidence and guidance given. Their 2009 patient information leaflet aims to provide a concise summary of PMS, and summarize these guidelines for patients.

This book aims to help anyone wanting to know more about PMS, whatever the nature and severity of their symptoms – those who suffer with PMS themselves, and healthcare professionals or friends and family who want to understand it and its treatment better. It is for those who suffer with mild symptoms and want to know what lifestyle changes they can make that are actually shown to make a difference. It is for those who want to understand what's happening in their body during the monthly cycle and why they feel the way they do. Chapter 8 on severe PMS specifically addresses those women who suffer debilitating symptoms and may feel that they've tried everything to no avail. We make suggestions and outline the current evidence and recommendations for different complaints.

We cannot provide all the answers, and do not guarantee any magic cures, but we do believe knowledge is power, and so we aim to empower women with the knowledge they need to understand their bodies, their PMS, and the evidence (or sometimes lack of evidence) for the different ways to manage PMS.

In this book we endeavour to help women not just to survive but to find the best way for them to cope positively with PMS and make a real difference in their own lives. We hope to help women overcome premenstrual syndrome, appreciate their femininity and start enjoying life to the full.

We have done our utmost to represent accurately the best available evidence surrounding the history, symptoms and treatment of PMS. We cannot accept responsibility for any omissions, or the effect of treatments discussed.

Summary

- PMS includes a wide variety of symptoms and severity.
- Most women are affected in some way.
- Between 5 and 10 per cent of women have devastating symptoms.
- We aim to inform, empower and help all those affected directly or indirectly by PMS.

2

A history of PMS

Women have always been having babies, and consequently have always had periods. But have they really always felt as rough as we might during the week before? Have women suffered in silence for centuries and been ignored until the last few years?

The menstrual cycle has been known about since ancient times, and its association with fertility was not only understood but sometimes even celebrated (see for example the story of the goddess Hera below). Although the idea of premenstrual symptoms is a relatively new one, there are records of physical and mental symptoms related to the menstrual cycle from many different eras throughout history.

While most of us have had some kind of sex education and have learnt about periods at school, the idea of a monthly cycle and what causes it is one that has significantly developed over the years. Theories range from the Renaissance idea that the period is a 'purging' of all the junk that accumulates in a woman's body during the month (the more junk, the worse the purge) to seeing it as a release of an excess of pure blood that would have otherwise been needed for pregnancy and breastfeeding. There is writing from the seventeenth century describing essentially the same symptoms as we associate with PMS today – headaches, lethargy, 'heaviness', pains, swelling of the abdomen, and breast swelling and tenderness. These symptoms are ascribed to the swollen womb being essentially too full of blood, and causing trouble until it can be released. However, although medically recognized, it is unclear whether this was a socially accepted complaint, or that the seventeenth-century lady of the manor might be excused her hectic social schedule on such grounds.

The modern concept of PMT (premenstrual tension) was first proposed by R. T. Frank in 1931, and the idea of a real, medical condition, in which some women experience disabling premenstrual physical and psychological symptoms, began to be formally recognized by western society as a whole. In 1953 Dr Katharina Dalton suggested the term PMS (premenstrual syndrome) rather than PMT, as the premenstrual symptoms described by it relate to more than just tension. From the first suggestion of the existence of PMT it still took 50 years for much interest to be shown in the concept by the general public; media interest was sparked in the 1980s when it was proposed as a legal defence for acts of assault in a few high-profile cases. In today's commercial society, where sanitary towels are advertised everywhere from billboards to advert breaks on TV, there is less and less taboo around the whole subject and 'hormones' are becoming a more acceptable explanation for certain symptoms and feelings, although not necessarily always in a helpful way.

Attitudes towards PMS today vary widely across different cultures, generations and groups of people. While there are still those who would even debate its existence and validity as a condition, others would consider it unacceptable, taboo, or distasteful to discuss any symptoms relating to the menstrual cycle. The menstruating woman may be esteemed and considered to be delicate – worthy of respect and care; conversely others might consider her unclean and unable to participate in social or religious activities where she would cause 'contamination'.

Ancient attitudes

The existence of the woman's monthly cycle has been openly recognized for over 4,000 years. The relation of the moon to the monthly cycles has been recognized since ancient times; hence the term 'menstrual cycle' literally means 'moon cycle'. The moon was a symbol for both femininity and menstruation, associated with the new life that depends on women's cycles. Some ancient creation stories link the monthly blood-flow to the origins of life and the universe itself. The ancient veneration of women associated with these ideas has become a subject of much interest in recent years, especially sparked by such books as Dan Brown's *The Da Vinci Code* which discusses them in a fictional context.

In Ancient Greece the goddess Hera was celebrated as the goddess of menstruation. One of the festivals of her worship and celebration involved women gathering together at the time of the new moon, bathing and celebrating their blood-flow in a circle of lygos branches. They called on Hera to encourage their menstrual flow, purifying them and renewing their fertility. It seems that at this time menstruation was seen as a very positive event to be celebrated and shared, such that even if there were symptoms preceding it the focus was probably on preparing for this purifying process and celebration.

In early biblical times the monthly period was referred to as a time of uncleanness. Jewish law excused women from various religious practices, and anything from a person to a cushion touched by a menstruating woman was considered ceremonially unclean. It was forbidden to sleep with a woman during her period – in almost the same breath as forbidding sacrificing your children or having incestuous relationships with your sister.

The Qur'an shows a similar view to the ancient Jewish texts; when Muhammad is questioned about women's monthly cycles his response is first that it is an 'illness' or 'harmful' (depending on which translation you use) and second that men should not be sleeping with women during that time because they're 'unclean' and possibly potentially unsafe. It has been argued that the difference between this and the Jewish idea of uncleanness is that Muhammad doesn't say that the woman can't touch anything and will contaminate everything around her, only that it would be harmful for a man to sleep with her at that time. However, in practice, Islamic tradition forbids menstruating women from observing religious practices, including praying, fasting and touching the holy Qur'an, in much the same way as in Judaism.

An ancient Roman text confirms the negative view of menstruation, suggesting that a menstruating woman will make seeds sterile and plants will die if she touches them. This does not appear to be related to any religious view, but is stated almost as an observation, and is a belief that is still shared by certain cultures today. For example, some people in India would still maintain that for whatever reason, food goes off more quickly if a woman prepares it at the wrong time of the month – a worrying concept if you are the only woman of the house and your husband can't pitch in with the cooking when you're on ...

Theories have been proposed that these religious regulations are/ were to protect women at their most vulnerable time from extra religious and marital duties and allow them 'space'. However, there is little or no mention of this justification in religious writings. The Bible even records Rachel using her period as a sneaky way to avoid standing up during a house search, so that she could hide some forbidden family idols – not a story to boost sympathy for women's vulnerability! The concept of symptoms preceding the monthly period, rather than related to the uncleanness during the time of bleeding, appears to be relatively new, and is not mentioned in these texts.

How have attitudes developed?

It seems that the 'unclean' view of menstruation persisted for hundreds of years, no less so than in the hyper-religious Victorian era. In Victorian times women were seen as clean and pure, and their bodies were considered as temples, probably in reference to biblical terms. They were not to destroy the purity of their bodies with excessive jewellery, unwomanly physical exertion or any other activity that might contaminate them. Given that women were expected to work hard at running their strict households, almost like military operations, it seems likely that there was little time for such a concept as PMS to be considered as a disease entity. Interestingly, the idea of women suffering from 'hysteria' was reasonably widely accepted, and may actually have referred to those emotional symptoms caused by PMS, but just blamed on women being women and generally a bit overemotional at times (quite a well-accepted phenomenon!).

There is some reference made to menstrual symptoms in medical writings from the time. For example, Sir Henry Maudsley wrote in 1874 about women being basically incapacitated for at least one week of the month, commenting on the emotional and physical 'derangement' caused by the ovarian cycle. In the nineteenth century the idea developed and grew that hormones from the ovaries were the major cause of women's complaints, from 'menstrual madness' and hysterical vomiting to nymphomania and masturbation. At this time surgery was just taking off, and the concept of removing a woman's ovaries to 'cure' all such problems was developed, with several reports of success.

There is also reference to 'puerperal mania' during that time. This suggested that women effectively lose their sanity for a while after giving birth, becoming irrational and emotional in much the same way as they might in the premenstrual phase. This phenomenon would now be described as postnatal depression or puerperal psychosis. It may be that this puerperal madness (blamed on the traumatic events of pregnancy and childbirth) was more socially acceptable than simply menstrual symptoms, although we can only speculate.

In the mid to late nineteenth century entrepreneur Lydia Pinkham of Massachusetts believed that some women suffer from specific disorders, including some related to menstruation. She invented and marketed a famous medicinal cocktail to help with many different illnesses in men and women alike ('Lydia E. Pinkham's Vegetable Compound'), with a marketing thrust towards women. She published a 'Private Text-Book upon Ailments Peculiar to Women', aimed at treating those ailments that affect women specifically, and invited women to write to her company for advice on various menstrual and other disorders. She clearly had her business head well screwed on, aiming to advocate and sell as much as possible of her potion – and was very successful at it. Her product is one of the best-known medicines of the time and similar products today still rely on her name's advertising power. She seems to have been a pioneer of empowering women with knowledge about their bodies and the information around menstrual symptoms that we have always wanted but often still don't get.

In the USA leaflets about menstruation for pubertal girls began to be produced from the 1920s onwards by companies such as Kotex: for example, 'Marjorie May's Twelfth Birthday'. It has been suggested that the idea of purification through menstruation was promoted by the advertising industry, and this is certainly the case in this particular leaflet, which is not at all subtle in its advertising stance. In it Marjorie May's mother explains to her the basics of a menstrual period. The leaflet unashamedly describes Kotex towels as far superior to any others, and leaves Marjorie May almost excited about starting her 'new purification', which will make her feel 'quite a young lady'! The aim was to make what had been a very taboo subject throughout the Victorian era much more universally acceptable.

As menstruation became more widely understood and discussed in the public arena, the advertising focus was on reinforcing it in a positive light – presumably with the aim of making sanitary protection more acceptable and therefore more profitable. Leaflets from the 1960s for young girls aim to affirm menstruation as a positive event, establishing the beginning of womanhood. For example, 'It's Time You Knew' by Tampax (1966) mentions 'pre-menstrual "blues"' and makes various suggestions including dietary changes (essentially the same advice as we would give today), exercise and attitude, as well as keeping a menstrual diary and consulting your doctor if necessary. As the concept of menstruation and the need for support with issues relating to it became more acceptable, adverts for sanitary protection became more widespread throughout the 1960s; they now comprise an industry worth billions of pounds.

In recent years PMS has been used as a legal defence for many criminal cases from burglary to assault and child abuse. One study suggested that as many as half of crimes committed by women take place in the four days before their periods start, giving good backing for PMS as a cause of crime. Media and public interest soared in 1981 when two women accused of murder had their convictions seriously reduced because their PMS was considered so severe that it made them effectively mad enough to kill without being responsible for their actions. Christine English lost her cool with her lover and deliberately rammed him with her car, killing him. She told police that she was suffering from PMS and already angry at him, so when he showed her the middle finger it was the last straw and she simply lost control and snapped. The courts accepted this, and let her off a custodial sentence. In the same year Sandie Craddock stabbed a workmate to death after a fight, claiming her PMS had made her lose control. When the courts reviewed how her many previous acts of violence and convictions were related to her menstrual cycle the charge against her was reduced and she was excused prison – instead being ordered to take progesterone.

In the 1970s and 1980s there was widespread concern that PMS would be used as an excuse for every crime and that the courts would be inundated by women who wanted to blame their hormones for all their criminal misdemeanours. Fortunately this doesn't seem to have happened, and although it is likely that in rare cases PMS, or PMDD (premenstrual dysphoric disorder), is indeed so severe that women are led to act in ways that are not only totally out of character but also socially and legally unacceptable, it seems that the justice system has kept a reasonable perspective on this. Nevertheless, accepting such a plea does leave us with the question of what to do with women in such situations. Because their 'insanity' is only present for probably a quarter of the month or less it's not really reasonable to lock them up in mental hospitals. But then we have the question of whether they are likely to re-offend next month. Some courts have suggested progesterone therapy as 'rehabilitation'; others have prescribed counselling or 'medical help'. There doesn't seem to be an easy answer, other than trying to help sufferers before their symptoms become so bad as to make them lose control completely.

Cultural differences in attitudes today

It is difficult, and not always very helpful, to stereotype a single view to any particular cultural group. However, we can learn a lot from looking at our differences, including the different ways PMS is viewed and how women suffering from it may be treated.

In certain parts of the world menarche (the time of a girl's first period) is seen as a significant event involving celebrations, sometimes even lasting for days. For example, in Arapesh society in New Guinea, a girl becomes the centre of a great ceremony when she first menstruates. She has nettles rubbed all over her, including in the vagina, fasts for up to a week and then has decorative cuts sliced into her skin by her uncle. All this sounds like serious torture (and probably feels like it at the time) but is apparently a way of celebrating her entry into womanhood. A more enjoyable way to come of age might be the South Indian/Sri Lankan ceremony where a girl sits on banana leaves, has a special ginger drink containing raw eggs, and then gets bathed in milk before having a family feast. It's probably best not to try and imagine what a mess might be produced with all that milk at such a time of the month. The point is that even today, in parts of the world, reaching womanhood is seen as a thing of wonder. Perhaps our negative-thinking society would benefit from some of the positivity that can be associated with a woman's monthly cycle.

There are few specific religious or cultural views on PMS itself. Although certain religions state that a woman is unclean during her period, with specific restrictions at that time, prior to bleeding there are few beliefs or customs. Buddhists would see PMS as a part of nature – the same way as any other ailment – and advocate the use of meditation to ease premenstrual symptoms. New Age followers would generally accept the existence of PMS and attribute it to hormonal or energy imbalances or toxins from which women need to be cleansed. Some would even suggest that PMS is a result of menstruation being unsuccessful at ridding the body of toxins from the womb, in the same way that irritable bowel syndrome (IBS) has been proposed as resulting from too many toxins in the gut. The scientific evidence for this theory is certainly limited, but it is an interesting idea. Numerous alternative remedies are advocated, such as homoeopathy, aromatherapy, herbal medicines and crystal therapies. Although the cynic would say that it's because they want to make money from you, alternative practitioners or followers of New Age-type thinking may often sadly be far more attentive and sympathetic than your GP or those in more conventional medicine.

The taboo

The widespread advertising and availability of sanitary protection is a testament to how far we have come as a society: from shunning a woman on her period as unclean, to accepting that it is a normal part of life that we all have to deal with. Nevertheless, despite the society-wide visibility of Tampax products in adverts and virtually all public toilets, the message is still more about discretion – the smaller the tampon pack, the more it looks like a lipstick case or anything other than what it is, the better. There will always be arguments from über-feminists that this is wrong and that it should be acceptable to whack your superabsorbents out on the dinner table before you head to the bathroom, just as there are those who totally disagree with exposing young children to products that they need to know nothing about before they reach puberty themselves (and men who think it's just 'gross'!).

However, there is a huge difference between accepting the general idea of menstruation as a part of life, and showing understanding to those of us who genuinely suffer prior to our periods, when we may not have much to show for it all. At least when you're on your period you can justify feeling rubbish because you can see that you're bleeding and there's something physically going on. When you know you're due, can't even pour a cup of tea without crying because you overfilled the mug, and feel like you're hiding America's nuclear weapon store inside your bloated tum, its not so easy to blame it on anything physical and much easier to feel that you're just hopeless at coping. Especially when the media only deals with the time of your period – we haven't seen many high-profile adverts on beating the blues and joining in the sexy netball games or parties during your menstrual pro-drome.

Perhaps it's because it's so easy to attribute all these symptoms to feminine weakness (why can't she pull herself together?), or perhaps it's because women themselves like to attribute all weaknesses to 'hormone trouble', as if this absolves them of the responsibility of being in a simple grump. This often leaves all those women who really need help reluctant to ask for it, even from their GPs. Perhaps we need a chlamydia-style public health campaign to wake society up to the fact that thousands of women genuinely are suffering, and show people that (a) it's OK to ask for help, and (b) there is help available at many different levels, from slight life-style modifications to alternative therapies or dramatic treatments for very severe cases.

Some critics have suggested that promoting awareness of PMS might lead to irresponsible women adding it to their list of accept-able complaints to call in sick with on a Monday morning. There will always be people who will abuse trust, say that they are sick when they're not and try to take advantage of others' misfortune – but this is surely no reason to leave a huge number of women struggling in misunderstood silence.

Some would argue that the labelling and medicalization of PMS leaves women feeling that their bodies are somehow dysfunctional or broken, making us feel angry, guilty or disgusted with ourselves and our bodies. However, the first step to solving the problem of premenstrual symptoms is to acknowledge them, and then search for a solution, which may or may not be medical – as we will later discuss.

The taboo of menstruation, and particularly of PMS, makes it a suitable topic for jokes in today's society where often the greater a taboo, the more mileage there is to be had from it. There are plenty of sexual jokes relating to menstruation, and all of us will be familiar with the understanding look and sometimes less than subtle sniggers when Jane slams the lid of the photocopier or snaps at someone in the office – 'must be the wrong time of the month' (whether she's like it every day of the month or not). While we may join in these jokes as much as the next girl (or guy), we're not really helping our cause by reinforcing men's perception that we are indeed the weaker sex, subject to hormones that turn us into demons every month.

In reality these hormones do not have to control us, and some women do report positive premenstrual symptoms such as a better mood, increased creativity or boosted sex drive; perhaps we should actually be able to celebrate those monthly changes that may make us more sensitive or in touch with our emotions in a positive way, embracing what it means to be a woman, rather than accepting our lot as victims. Just beware that in this imperfect world storming in to remind the lads that their jokes aren't helpful may make them think it's the wrong time of the month for you too, resulting in more laughter than understanding.

Nevertheless, whatever the views and taboos of those around us, PMS certainly needs to be recognized and treated to stop women suffering. Over the centuries the idea that women's femininity and fertility are positive – to be valued and even celebrated – has been largely lost, especially in western society. We as women need to take the lead in appreciating and celebrating our femininity, understanding our bodies and overcoming those things that take the fun out of being a woman. This book aims to help and encourage you to do that.

Summary

- Fertility, menstruation and the monthly cycle have been known about for thousands of years.
- Women have been both celebrated and seen as unclean.
- Some Victorians attributed symptoms to hormones and removed ovaries as a cure for 'monthly madness'.
- The idea of premenstrual syndrome has developed over the last 50 years, even being used as a legal defence.
- Although menstruation is now widely understood there is still some taboo and controversy surrounding PMS.

3

The normal menstrual cycle

What is actually going on inside a woman every month?

Hormones

Let's start with the basics. Often we talk about blaming everything on our hormones, and hormones being muddled and making us feel rubbish. But first things first: what are hormones and what hormones are we talking about?

Hormones are literally chemical messengers in the body that send messages from one organ in the body to another, for example from the brain to the kidneys, the gut or the womb. There are steroid hormones (fat-based) or non-steroid hormones (protein-based). We all have some of each, and steroid hormones don't necessarily equate to the kind of hormones that make body-builders big, butch and aggressive (anabolic steroids). Hormones can do all sorts of things, from telling your kidneys to conserve water and stop producing so much urine, to telling your breasts to start producing milk ready for a baby. Sex hormones are the ones specifically related to reproduction and contributing to the physical differences between men and women. The main sex hormones are oestrogen, progesterone and testosterone.

The normal menstrual cycle

The hormones that we're interested in are those that are involved in the menstrual cycle. The menstrual cycle refers to the monthly pattern of bleeding and ovulation that naturally occurs in women. Menarche is the name for the time a girl has her first period, and menopause is the name for the time when periods cease. The normal menstrual cycle lasts for about 28 days, give or take a few days in different women. For some women it is as regular as clockwork, while for others it might be 28 days one month, 20 another month, and 40 the next. On the whole, the cycle is likely to be longer when you're younger, get shorter as you get older, and become somewhat erratic and irregular in the last year or few years before you reach menopause, which is on average around the age of 51 in the western world. If you have a hysterectomy (removal of the womb) before this you will stop having periods and so technically have an early menopause, although if your ovaries have not been removed at the same time as the womb they may continue to work and produce hormones until about the age at which you would have reached the menopause naturally.

Phases of the menstrual cycle

On a very basic level, the menstrual cycle can be divided into two phases: the *follicular* and *luteal* phases. The cycle begins with vaginal bleeding (menstruation) which lasts for between two and seven days in most women. You can think of this as a clearing of the lining of the womb (called the endometrium), ready to start afresh and prepare for the possibility of pregnancy.

This phase, up until the point of ovulation, is known as the follicular phase. After menstruation, the lining of the womb slowly starts to grow again, and in one of the ovaries, an egg begins to emerge (usually just one, but it can be more) from the collection of eggs waiting to develop. Initially a few follicles (each containing an egg) in the ovary are stimulated to grow, hence the name follicular phase. After a short time one particular follicle predominates and the others seemingly give up. The follicle grows for about a week, until a surge of specific hormones causes it to burst open, releasing the egg from the follicle around it. This is the event known as ovulation.

The egg that is released is called an oocyte. The egg is now free and fit to be fertilized, and is moved from the ovary along the fallopian tubes and into the womb, where it hopes to meet an engaging sperm. If there has recently been some unprotected sex, and there are sperm around, one lucky sperm may break through the surface layer of the egg, fertilizing it. The two will then become one, implanting into the nice soft lining of the womb that has been

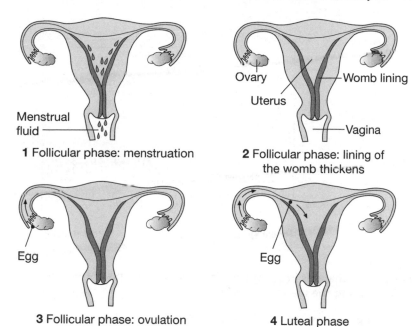

1 Follicular phase: menstruation

2 Follicular phase: lining of the womb thickens

3 Follicular phase: ovulation

4 Luteal phase

Figure 3.1 Phases of the menstrual cycle

growing for them and developing into an embryo and eventually a baby.

The second half of the cycle, after ovulation, is the luteal phase. The name luteal comes from the fact that the key player in this process, as opposed to the follicle in the first phase, is now a structure that is officially called the *corpus luteum*. (This literally means 'yellow body', so think of it as a bit like the yoke of an egg, although technically it is not part of the egg.) The corpus luteum is the remains of the empty follicle which is left after the follicle from the first phase has burst, and the egg has gone off on its travels towards the womb. The corpus luteum, being left behind, gets to work at producing hormones to help the egg in case it is fertilized and needs to implant in the endometrium, the lining of the womb. During this time, more blood vessels grow in the endometrium and it grows thicker and softer, ready to support an embryo.

If the egg is not fertilized the corpus luteum breaks down and disintegrates. At the same time, the lining of the womb becomes

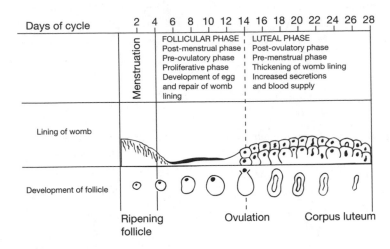

Figure 3.2 Changes in the womb lining and development of the follicle during the menstrual cycle

too thick to support itself, and starts to break down and shed – causing a new period to start. It is nearly always exactly 14 days between ovulation and menstruation. So if your periods are regular you can predict exactly when you will ovulate and menstruate; but if they are irregular you can't, as the time between menstruation and the next ovulation often varies. You will ovulate and be most fertile exactly 14 days before your next period is due, which in a regular 28-day cycle will be Day 14, if Day 1 is the first day of your period. If you have a regular 32-day cycle, you will ovulate on Day 18.

To avoid any confusion with what you might have read elsewhere, the follicular phase is sometimes known as the proliferative phase (in reference to the proliferation and growth of the endometrium) or the preparatory phase (in reference to the preparation for ovulation). The second half of the cycle, the luteal phase, is sometimes referred to as the secretory phase (in reference to the endometrium becoming thicker and producing some secretions), or the waiting phase (waiting to see if an embryo appears in the womb). To keep things simple they are just referred to here as the follicular and luteal phases, although it may be helpful to be aware of their other names.

You may already know all this, but it is important to be clear in our minds about what is going on in the reproductive cycle, so that we can understand the role of the hormones involved and how they can be disrupted, causing us problems. This also helps when people start blaming things on high or low oestrogen or progesterone levels – if you understand the basics it's harder to be fooled by people trying to sound scientific and sell you something when they don't have a clue.

Changing hormones

We can now talk about what hormones have to do with the whole process. The three main sex hormones are oestrogen (or estrogen if you're American), progesterone and testosterone. These are all steroid hormones, which means that they are fat-based, and fat-soluble. Testosterone is more important in men – there is not much testosterone around in women, so the main hormones we're concerned with are oestrogen and progesterone.

There are various forms of these hormones in the body, and various versions of them are found in different medications. The most important type of oestrogen is oestrodiol (or estrodiol) which is produced by the ovaries and also by the placenta and, in men, in the testes. Progesterone is the most important of a group of hormones, progestogens, and is produced in the ovaries, the brain and the placenta. There are numerous types of man-made progestogens, and these are discussed in Chapter 7 in relation to hormone therapies.

There are three main headquarters in the body involved in the regulation and production of these hormones – two in the brain and one in the ovaries. In the brain a small gland called the hypothalamus detects various levels of chemicals in the blood, and releases hormones that travel to another small gland called the pituitary, telling it to release other hormones. This interaction is known as the hypothalamic–pituitary axis, and is crucial to regulating the monthly cycle of events in the body. The hormones from the pituitary in turn act on the ovaries, and result in production of the hormones we're interested in – oestrogen and progesterone. Just to confuse matters, it's worth bearing in mind that oestrogen is also found elsewhere in the body, and since it is a fat-based hormone, it is produced in fatty tissues, such that women who are overweight are likely to have more 'peripheral' (that is, out there in the skin layers and fatty tissues) oestrogen than skinny women. It's unclear what effect this extra oestrogen has on PMS.

During your normal monthly cycle, there is a pattern of change in hormone levels which is important, and the changes are probably more important than the absolute levels themselves.

If we start at the top and work down, we begin with the hypothalamic–pituitary axis. The pituitary releases two particular hormones, called gonadotrophins – first, luteinizing hormone (LH), and second, follicle-stimulating hormone (FSH). Both of these basically do what they say on the tin, as we will see in a moment. The hypothalamus kicks off the whole process by releasing short bursts of gonadotrophin-releasing hormone (GnRH), which causes the pituitary to release those gonadotrophins. Initially in the cycle both oestrogen and progesterone levels are low.

GnRH causes release of LH and FSH from the pituitary gland. The FSH does its job by stimulating follicles in the ovary, and a few follicles start to develop. As these follicles grow, they each begin to produce small amounts of oestrogen around the area of the ovary, which then gets into the bloodstream. Various mechanisms prevent a muddle of too many follicles, and so one follicle emerges stronger than the rest, and takes on the task of producing oestrogen for all of them while the rest go back to their places and rest again. During this time the levels of oestrogen in the blood gradually rise as it is produced by initially several and then one specific follicle in the ovary. Progesterone levels stay low in the first half of the cycle.

The gonadotrophins LH and FSH keep on being produced by the pituitary during this follicular stage, until a point just before ovulation where the pituitary stops producing FSH, and makes one last big spurt of LH. This sudden increase in luteinizing hormone does what it says – it causes the main follicle to burst, releasing the oocyte, or egg, which is now ready to be fertilized, and producing that 'yellow body', the corpus luteum. Ovulation – the release of the egg and the production of the corpus luteum – begins the luteal phase of the cycle.

Normal premenstrual changes

The luteal phase is, of course, the phase that we're most interested in when we talk about PMS, because it is the time leading up to menstruation – the point when your symptoms occur. After ovulation the egg is fertile for only about 24 hours. The accepted time of most fertility – when the egg is most amenable to fertilization by a sperm – is Days 12–16. A sperm can survive for up to four days inside a woman's body, and therefore intercourse during this time has the greatest potential to result in pregnancy. Of course, you can never be certain of the time of ovulation until it has happened, so if ovulation occurred earlier or later than usual you could potentially still get pregnant at other times; this is why you cannot rely on timings alone for contraception.

If the egg was fertilized it would need progesterone (literally the 'pro-pregnancy' hormone) as well as oestrogen to help it grow and establish itself. Because the embryo is initially too small to produce enough progesterone for itself, the body produces progesterone in the second half of the cycle to help out any embryo that might be growing. If an embryo is present and begins to develop, the growing placenta will later take over production of progesterone to keep the pregnancy going, but until this point the hormone comes from a separate source – the corpus luteum.

As the corpus luteum doesn't know whether or not the egg has been fertilized, it has to give it the benefit of a doubt, and act as if fertilization had occurred. It therefore produces progesterone and oestrogen to help support any embryo that might emerge. After exactly 14 days the corpus luteum has had enough, and dies. At the same time, if the lining of the womb, which has been growing and thickening, has not had any signals to indicate that a pregnancy is present it starts to break down. This marks the end of the luteal phase, and menstruation begins.

In the time between ovulation and menstruation, oestrogen and progesterone levels rise in the blood as they are released by the corpus luteum. The combination of these hormones acts on the hypothalamus and stops it from producing GnRH. The gonadotrophins (LH and FSH) therefore stop being produced by the pituitary gland; as there is the possibility of a pregnancy developing there is now no need to stimulate other follicles to ovulate.

Progesterone levels are low in the first half of the cycle, and increase after ovulation, with a peak at about Day 21. There are two surges in oestrogen levels. The first is in the follicular phase, as it is being produced by the developing follicle, with a surge around Days 7–14 – just before the surge of LH that triggers ovulation. Oestrogen temporarily falls, then the second surge is around Day 21, at which point the progesterone levels are also high. Progesterone levels start to rise as soon as ovulation occurs, stay relatively high for a bit longer than the oestrogen levels, and don't drop so much until the last few days of the cycle. Therefore in the premenstrual phase (the week before menstruation) you will have quite low oestrogen levels, while progesterone levels are higher and just begin to drop in the last day or two of the cycle. This is best understood by looking at the graph in Figure 3.3 which shows the changing hormone levels.

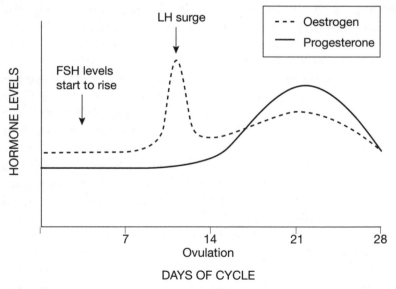

Figure 3.3 Hormone changes during the menstrual cycle

What effects do these hormones have?

Some of the natural functions of oestrogen and progesterone and the importance of these in menstruation, pregnancy and family planning are described here to help your understanding of what's going on in your body, and particularly what's normal. The relation of these hormones to the emotional and physical symptoms of PMS is discussed in Chapters 5 and 6.

Progesterone

Progesterone causes a number of changes in the body that would help it to support a pregnancy. It causes smooth muscle in the body to relax. Smooth muscle is not the same as the muscle in your arms or legs that might get tense or stiff, so this relaxation is not quite as desirable as it sounds. This is a type of muscle that you don't have voluntary control over, and is found in the womb (the myometrium), in blood vessels and also in the gut. These effects are important in pregnancy as they help not only in allowing the womb to relax and prepare for a growing baby, but also in exerting a relaxing effect on the walls of blood vessels, which helps the body to cope with the extra volume of blood in later pregnancy.

Unfortunately, when progesterone rises it also causes the muscle in your gut to relax. While this might help you to absorb as much goodness as possible from your food, it can lead to constipation, nausea and bloating – common symptoms in pregnancy and also PMS. Progesterone also affects what goes into your digestive system; it increases your appetite and tells your body to switch into fat-storage mode. This is crucial in the first few weeks of pregnancy to provide plenty of energy and nutrients for later on as a baby increases its demands on the mother's body.

One of the most important roles of progesterone is in helping the lining of the womb to become softer and more suitable for implantation of an embryo. Insufficient progesterone can cause or contribute to infertility, and so it is sometimes given in fertility treatment in order to help the endometrium prepare for pregnancy. In vitro fertilization (IVF) treatment involves the woman taking progesterone even after the embryo is implanted into the womb, as the body isn't able to produce enough naturally for an unnaturally conceived pregnancy.

This may seem a bit confusing, as progestogens are also used for contraception, to prevent pregnancy. However, the key is when and how progestogen is given. In the context of contraception, enough progestogen is given for the hypothalamus to detect it and therefore stop secreting GnRH. This means that LH and FSH are not secreted by the pituitary gland, and the hormone cycle is suppressed, thereby preventing ovulation. Even on the days off the pill (the seven-day pill break) there is not a long enough break from progestogen for the body to revert to its normal cycle, so although there will be some 'menstrual' bleeding as some of the lining of the womb sheds, there is no actual ovulation taking place, and therefore very little chance of pregnancy.

On the other hand, in the context of helping with fertility, progesterone is taken only in the luteal phase of the cycle (after ovulation) to help boost the growth and preparation of the lining of the womb for pregnancy implantation. In this situation it does not interfere with ovulation, since this has already taken place, and therefore the progesterone is helping to boost the natural hormone changes that should be going on anyway, rather than trying to stop them.

Another helpful role of progesterone is its effect on body temperature, which is useful for women who want to identify when they ovulate for the purposes of trying to conceive by natural family planning methods. This is discussed in Chapter 6.

Oestrogen

Oestrogen contributes to growth of breast tissue and endometrial tissue. Therefore, if given in the wrong way over a long period of time, it can increase the possibility of breast cancer and endometrial cancer. Progesterone regulates the effects of oestrogen on these tissues, which is why it is given in combination with oestrogen in hormone replacement therapy (HRT) or the combined oral contraceptive pill (COCP) in order to reduce the risk of these cancers.

During the normal cycle, the endometrium grows much thicker initially while just oestrogen is acting on it, and when progesterone gets involved in the second half of the cycle the tissue stops growing thicker but grows in a different way, becoming more vascular, softer, and producing more secretions to help with implantation.

Oestrogen has an important effect on the body's metabolism of calcium, increasing uptake of calcium into the bones, therefore making them stronger. This is believed to be the main reason why older women are much more likely than older men to suffer from broken bones (fractures). The levels of oestrogen in the bloodstream drop dramatically after a woman stops menstruating (at the time of menopause), thus reducing the uptake of calcium into the bones and making them progressively weaker and more prone to fractures as she gets older.

Oestrogen may cause your body to retain water and salt. It increases blood-flow to the uterus. It may also reduce movement of food along the gut, acting in addition to progesterone to contribute to constipation and bloating.

Certain proteins in the body may be affected by oestrogen. Collagen is one of the proteins that gives strength and firmness to different bodily tissues, and has been made famous by being artificially implanted or injected in plastic surgery procedures, particularly in the lips. It is believed that oestrogen may boost the production of collagen in certain body tissues, possibly increasing their strength and firmness. This may well be why after the menopause some women using hormone replacement therapy (HRT), which contains oestrogen, report an improvement in their skin and hair, since these tissues appear to be stronger with the increased oestrogen levels. A recent study showed that oestrogen cream may boost collagen production in skin that is not sun-damaged, making it firmer and therefore reducing wrinkles.

Some collagen fibres may be triggered to loosen or relax by changing hormone levels, such as in pregnancy, and one effect of this is on the collagen holding together some of the ligaments in the pelvis. This slightly loosens the pelvis towards the end of a pregnancy and helps the baby's head to pass through the pelvis for a natural birth. The effect of the lower levels of oestrogen outside of pregnancy on collagen is unknown, but the premenstrual fall in oestrogen levels might contribute to aches and pains in the body as ligaments around certain joints relax.

Finally, the natural vaginal mucus is significantly affected by changing hormone levels during the menstrual cycle. While oestrogen is steadily increasing in the follicular phase, it causes the mucus secretions produced by the cervix to become thin and alkaline, as you will notice in the first half of your cycle. After ovulation, when progesterone is more predominant, the natural mucus discharge from the vagina becomes much thicker and slightly more acidic. This is again helpful to women who want to use natural family planning methods to identify where they're at in the cycle, either to try to conceive or to avoid pregnancy.

Summary

- Hormones are chemical messengers in the body.
- Oestrogen and progesterone are important sex hormones in the menstrual cycle.
- Oestrogen and progesterone levels are low in the first (follicular) half of the cycle.
- Ovulation occurs around Day 14.
- Oestrogen levels peak around ovulation then fall temporarily.
- In the second (luteal) half of the cycle there is a smaller peak of oestrogen and progesterone is high until just before menstruation.

4

What is PMS?

Definition of PMS

Premenstrual syndrome by very definition means a syndrome of symptoms that occur premenstrually – that is, in the time before a period starts. A number of physical, emotional and psychological symptoms are reported within the spectrum of PMS, including abdominal cramps, headaches, breast tenderness, fatigue, irritability and a feeling of emotional instability, to name but a few. A total of over 150 symptoms have been reported as part of the syndrome, and the main key to diagnosis is not so much the nature of the symptoms but the timing of them. If you experience bloating and abdominal pains coming and going all the time, irrespective of the time of your monthly cycle, it is not PMS. Premenstrual symptoms occur during the week before your period, and resolve within a few days of starting your period.

In addition, you cannot have a diagnosis of PMS if you have only had one episode of symptoms. It has to be cyclical – symptoms should show a pattern of occurring before your period most months, if not every month. Some women report cyclical symptoms after they have had their womb removed but the ovaries have been left behind, as the ovaries are still producing a monthly pattern of changing hormones. Even though these women don't menstruate, they have the equivalent of PMS because it is monthly, and caused by the hormone changes that cause PMS.

Some women have symptoms for ten days, starting a week before and lasting for three days of their bleed. Others have symptoms for longer than this, or for only a few days before their period, or perhaps just on the first day of bleeding. Symptoms may be mild or totally debilitating; but if they fit into the premenstrual time-frame, they are classified as PMS. There is a recognized spectrum of severity of PMS, and this is discussed in depth in Chapter 8 on severe PMS.

Premenstrual dysphoric disorder (PMDD) is a term not much used by health professionals in the UK, but is commonly used in the USA to refer to severe PMS.

It is very important to note that every woman is different; just because someone you know complains of certain premenstrual symptoms, it does not mean that you are abnormal in having totally different symptoms. In fact, for some women the onset of abdominal cramps a few days before their period is a reassuring symptom, affirming that (a) their bodies are continuing to work as usual, and (b) they are not pregnant! Of course, for other women similar symptoms may be met with dread, as they signal the beginning of a week of being totally unable to function on any more than a very basic level. The effect on you of your premenstrual symptoms will depend on numerous factors such as the nature and severity of your symptoms themselves, your pain threshold, other health issues, and the support or stress levels in your environment.

There can be enormous pressure to feel 'normal': to experience the 'normal' symptoms that every woman has every month, and to relate to what everyone else experiences. It may feel acceptable to complain of disabling pains or migraines, but unthinkable to decline a client meeting because you know you may be so emotional at that time that you could end up crying into your coffee if it doesn't go well. Some women feel tearful, some irrational, some are ravenously hungry, some just lose their confidence and become quieter than usual. Some have such painful breasts that they can't bear to wear a bra, some have intolerable headaches, some get diarrhoea; others become violent and aggressive.

Numerous other less common symptoms have been reported. Some women hear voices in the premenstrual time, which resolve with menstruation, and worry that they have schizophrenia. Others become severely depressed and suicidal despite feeling fine at other times of the month. The message of this book is that whichever woman you are, or whoever you're reading this book to understand and support, PMS is really more normal than abnormal, and however it affects you, you are certainly not alone.

Diagnosis of PMS

PMS can be diagnosed clinically by recognizing that the symptoms you are affected by are indeed occurring in the premenstrual phase of your cycle. The best way to confirm this is to keep a diary of symptoms. While this may feel like a chore, in actual fact if you can just write a few words describing what symptoms you've experienced that day, or what has upset you, other important events or things you've eaten, and also noting when each period starts and finishes, after a couple of months you may be able to look back and see a pattern. This will help you to confirm whether or not it is PMS that is causing your symptoms, and to understand the nature and pattern of your symptoms. You may notice, for example, that your symptoms are much worse if you've had a number of takeaways the week before, or that during the months that you exercise, or meet up with supportive friends, you are much more able to cope. Understanding what affects your PMS can be a great motivator for making the changes you know you should but find hard to do.

Additionally, if you feel that you need to see a doctor or other professional about your symptoms it will be easier for you to demonstrate their premenstrual nature, and for the doctor to understand and suggest treatments, if you have a clear diary of your symptoms. The value of having a diary to show to a healthcare professional cannot be overestimated. It can also be tremendously helpful to look back and see the effect of different treatments.

For the purposes of research into treatments for PMS, different diagnostic tools have been designed to confirm that any medications tested are definitely treating the right women. The criteria for these generally involve a certain number of symptoms taken from a specific list, which must be experienced exclusively in the luteal or premenstrual phase. However, in real life, things are not always so clear cut. Since you may have only one symptom, which is very severe, or symptoms that are not all listed in the official criteria, it is better to rely on a diary to confirm the timing of your symptoms rather than try to fit yourself into one of these criteria-based models.

Why do some women get it and not others?

This is a question that has been asked by many women, healthcare workers and researchers, and the answer is sadly not as simple as we would like. Women of different ages, backgrounds, races and socio-economic groups are affected by PMS, and there seems to be a large number of potential contributing factors which cannot really be taken individually. These are discussed in more depth in Chapter 5. There is some evidence that certain families may have more women suffering with PMS than others, so if your mum has symptoms, then you and your sisters may well also be likely to, but even this is not certain.

Other risk factors include being significantly overweight, and smoking. It seems that women who smoke are more likely to develop PMS than those who don't; and the more you smoke and the longer you smoke for, the more likely you are to have symptoms.

Women who are classified as overweight or obese are also more likely to have PMS symptoms. One study found that a body mass index (BMI) of more than 30 made women three times more likely to suffer from PMS. The body mass index is calculated using a formula involving your weight and height, and can be obtained from charts and online calculators. Divide your weight (in kilograms) by the square of your height (in metres). An ideal BMI is between 20 and 25. A BMI of greater than 25 is considered overweight, and a person with a BMI of more than 30 is classified as obese.

It is believed that smoking and high body mass index may affect the hormone changes associated with PMS, and their effect on the body. If you smoke or are overweight you may find that you can reduce your PMS symptoms by addressing these issues.

'Pseudo-PMS'

You may feel that you are affected with far worse PMS than many of your girlfriends. On the other hand, you may find that you barely feel any different at all during the proverbial 'time of the month' in comparison to your friends who look like they're going through hell. So is it just down to pot luck, are some women more prone to

PMS than others? Or can we just blame it on our mothers and put it down to 'bad genes'?

One interesting study looked into the evolutionary model of PMS. It suggested that PMS tends to affect all women depending on what stage they're at in life. Apparently it all comes down to if and when women plan to have children. The study suggests that during the 'fertile' period – around the time of ovulation – women experience positive states in that they feel more confident in themselves in order to attract a 'mate' and for fertilization to follow. If this fails to occur then disappointment and frustration set in which manifest themselves as physical and emotional symptoms, or, PMS.

On the other hand, it was suggested that those women who have no desire to become pregnant, perhaps due to career reasons or simply because motherhood doesn't suit them at a particular time, tend to experience their 'PMS-like' symptoms during the fertile phase – at the time of ovulation. This is sometimes referred to as 'pseudo-PMS' since it does not actually occur premenstrually; and in contrast, these women tend to experience the heightened, positive states just before their period. This theory may be construed as portraying women as mere baby-making machines, but before you get offended, on a basic biological level, it could make some sense.

What PMS might be confused with

As already stressed, it is important to confirm that your symptoms are indeed premenstrual and not menstrual or occurring at another time in your cycle. For example, you may suffer from severe abdominal pains, which are cyclical, but not premenstrual. The pains could be due to ovulation, if they occur in the middle of your cycle (Mittelschmerz pains). These can be mild or severe, and last from hours to days, but are usually quite sharp pains on one side of the lower part of your tummy, occurring about 14 days before your period starts. Alternatively, the pains could be due to ovarian cysts; if they occur during your period, it could be endometriosis.

Your symptoms may in actual fact not be cyclical at all; it may be that although they bother you more premenstrually, when you record them in a diary those symptoms may occur intermittently throughout your cycle. You may find that you are blaming PMS for your stress and emotional problems, when in fact you are stressed or depressed all the time, and need to address the root cause. Abdominal pains, bloating, and intermittent diarrhoea and constipation could be caused by a number of different bowel problems including irritable bowel syndrome (IBS), although the symptoms of this may be worsened premenstrually. In any case, if you are troubled by symptoms that you may have thought were due to PMS, but having kept a diary you realize are not, you should see your doctor to find out what the cause really is – and get on top of it.

It is relatively common for certain medical disorders such as asthma, rheumatoid arthritis and epilepsy to be worsened around the premenstrual time. This is not actually PMS, and is known as 'premenstrual exaggeration' since although the symptoms are affected by menstruation, they exist at different times of the month as well. For example, migraine sufferers often report increased frequency or severity of their migraines around the time of their period. Although they may also suffer from different symptoms which are only present premenstrually, the migraines are not due to PMS, and should be treated as migraines. A doctor may suggest increasing preventative medication in the second half of the cycle to prevent this worsening, but this should be done under the supervision of the doctor treating the migraines, or whatever the relevant condition. Some people with epilepsy may have increased frequency of seizures around the time of their period, but again, while you may benefit from taking measures to treat PMS if you suffer from it in other ways, you should see your neurologist to discuss the timing of your seizures and treatment for them before you attribute it all to PMS.

Summary

- Premenstrual syndrome is defined as symptoms in the second half of the menstrual cycle.
- Diagnosis of PMS requires cyclical symptoms.
- A diary is very helpful for diagnosis and charting progress.
- Several symptoms may be attributed to PMS but are actually present throughout the cycle.
- Some medical conditions get worse premenstrually.
- It's best to see your doctor if you're worried about a diagnosis of PMS or another condition.

5

Emotional and psychological symptoms

PMS is characterized by a number of physical and psychological symptoms. One particular symptom may dominate over another and each symptom varies in severity from one individual to the next. In this chapter we explore how and why PMS can affect your mental well-being.

You may have been in a bad mood for no particular reason, become overly upset by the fact that your local supermarket ran out of your favourite brand of cereal bars, or felt paranoid that because the lady at the checkout didn't offer you help with your shopping this time she obviously has it in for you? How many times have you heard your partner, siblings, friends, colleagues (... the whole world!) say, 'Oh, it must be because it's her time of the month', 'She's just PMSing', or 'It must be her hormones!' Honestly, if I were given a pound ... !

When women voice genuine concerns or complaints during their premenstrual phase, it proves terribly frustrating for these concerns to be put down to 'feeling hormonal'. This simply heightens the angst and serves to delegitimatize their claims by shunning women as irrational, histrionic creatures – which of course we're not! So, ladies, on a positive note, at least we should be grateful that the world has acknowledged that there is something going on, on a monthly basis, that alters our behaviour, and that 'something' may be linked to our periods! Or is it? Can we really believe that our behaviour is down to our cycle? Well, the simple answer to that is yes.

Women experience a vast array of emotional and psychological symptoms around the time of their monthly cycle. These can be anything from slight irritability and low mood to severe depression or even complete psychosis. In this chapter we will talk about some of the most commonly reported symptoms, and try to make sense of why they occur.

Depression

During the monthly cycle women may experience anything from feeling a little low in mood to unbearable depression. It is important to distinguish between depression per se and depression being a specific symptom of PMS, as the management of it does vary. The simplest way to tell the difference is by looking at your pattern of mood. If depression occurs throughout the cycle and is relatively independent of where you are in your cycle then a diagnosis of depression is more likely. Women who already suffer with depression may find that their symptoms are exacerbated during their period. If, however, you find that you are experiencing depression during the luteal phase (following ovulation but just before your period is due) of your cycle each month, then your symptoms are more likely to be consistent with PMS.

In the following chapter we will look at how the physical symptoms associated with PMS, such as bloating and constipation, make us feel terrible. So, could it be that because we are experiencing all sorts of bodily injustices, we subsequently feel low in mood? After all, PMS or no PMS, anyone going through all those symptoms is bound to feel depressed, right? Could the fact that our hormones are whizzing around like there's no tomorrow and causing us to feel a little teary be the reason why we're more intolerant to physical discomforts, when on a 'normal' day we wouldn't really give a second thought to a bit of pain here and there? It's a bit like what came first, the chicken or the egg?

Well, bizarrely enough, it seems that they both come independently of one another. According to one study, the appearance of severe physical symptoms in the late luteal phase of the female reproductive cycle is not related to a worsening of psychological symptoms and it therefore concluded that psychological symptoms seem to be independent of the appearance of severe physical symptoms.

So, let's get down to the science bit! Serotonin, one of the body's 'feel-good' hormones, has a large number of roles. The complex interaction of our sex hormones – oestrogen and progesterone – affect the levels of serotonin (as well as some other chemicals) whizzing around in the part of the brain that is responsible for mood, emotions and behaviour: the limbic system.

Just to recap, oestrogen and progesterone travel in the bloodstream to various parts of the brain and it's the precise fluctuations of their levels that ensures that the menstrual cycle runs like clockwork. Oestrogen and progesterone receptors are abundant in the brain; the hormones travel easily from the bloodstream into the limbic system where they latch on to these receptors. Therefore, changes in these two hormone levels can directly affect the area of your brain controlling your mood, and change the way you feel. Oestrogen and progesterone levels have other effects too; for instance, in women with epilepsy, seizures are known to occur more frequently during times of high oestrogen levels (late follicular phase and ovulation) and they tend to decrease when progesterone levels are high.

Scientific evidence strongly suggests a link between depression and low levels of serotonin. Certain antidepressant medications, SSRIs (selective serotonin reuptake inhibitors), work by doing exactly the mechanism that they're named after: that is, inhibiting serotonin reuptake in the brain. They therefore exert their antidepressant effects by preventing the serotonin receptors in the brain from reabsorbing the circulating serotonin, thus ensuring that higher levels remain in the brain.

Monoamine oxidase (MAO) is a special protein found in the brain. One of its actions is to regulate the metabolism of serotonin, but what does that have to do with PMS? Well, oestrogens are known to block the action of MAO. This subsequently leads to higher serotonin levels as it is not broken down so much. Therefore there's more whizzing around in the brain to make you feel good, resulting in elevation of mood. Interestingly, therefore, it's not surprising that prescribing high-dose oestrogen to women suffering with depression has been explored with some success.

Progesterone has an opposite effect to oestrogen in that it increases the concentration of MAO in the brain. This means that there is more MAO to break down your happy hormone, serotonin, and bring down your mood with it. Progesterone is also believed to increase the activity of another chemical in the brain associated with anxiety and depression: gamma-aminobutyric acid (GABA). This, combined with the reduction in serotonin, may explain why you feel down or depressed in the week before your period, when progesterone levels peak.

This may sound complicated, and is in fact vastly more complicated still, but it can be broken down simply to the effects of changing serotonin levels in the brain: oestrogen increases it and progesterone decreases it.

Knowing all this, it is not surprising that treatment with progesterone alone, for example for contraceptive purposes, may lead to low mood and could worsen pre-existing depression in some women. It therefore makes sense to learn that the combination of oestrogen plus progesterone such as that used in birth control pills and menopausal hormone replacement therapy does not tend to worsen mood because the combined effects of the two hormones cancel each other out. The newer progesterones, discussed in Chapter 7, may have less effect in lowering serotonin.

During your time of the month, you may even make a conscious effort to try and appear happy and smiley in a vain attempt to offset your internal feelings. You try so hard to smile and laugh through your work colleagues' jokes (which really aren't that funny!) and fight off that incessant urge to burst out crying – until someone notices and asks, 'Is everything all right, you don't quite look yourself?', or 'Do you have that long face because you're on your period?' But just how did they know that?

Well, it seems that your face may be revealing much more to the world than you intend about what's really going on, despite your hardest efforts to conceal your true feelings. A recent study looked into the effects of PMS on facial expressions of sadness. It found that the activity of *musculus depressor anguli oris*, which is the anatomical name for the muscle responsible for causing our mouth to turn downwards (much like when we're sad), is increased during the luteal phase of the cycle, and therefore leads to 'subconscious frowning'!

Irritability and aggression

It may or may not be immediately obvious to you, but during your time of the month, one of the first behavioural changes that your partner/friends will notice about you is your irritability. Your behaviour may vary from developing a slight intolerance, to reducing those around you to tiptoeing around on eggshells for fear of having their heads bitten off for something relatively benign. If this is severe, you may feel constantly miserable and guilty as you see the effect of your aggression on those around you, but feel you can't control it.

Given that so far hormones are to be blamed for everything to do with PMS, which hormone is it this time that can cause a relatively sane person to fall off the edge into such an irrational state of emotional chaos? It's partly due to the action of oestrogen. At the time of ovulation (midway through your cycle), oestrogen levels are at their highest. Once ovulation has occurred, oestrogen levels begin to fall gradually. As we mentioned during the discussion on depression, oestrogen is important for raising serotonin levels (via MAO). Once oestrogen levels fall, so do serotonin levels, which leads to depressed mood and general grumpiness. It is therefore not surprising that you may be more irritable when you're feeling low.

In addition, the physical symptoms will not help matters. You may experience some tummy bloating which may cause your clothes to feel uncomfortable. Twinges and pain that accompany your period may also lower your 'irritability threshold'.

Other than hormones, there may be some deep-rooted psychological reasons causing increased irritability and frustration. Some psychologists have suggested that following ovulation, the ovum (the egg) is preparing to be fertilized and implanted into the womb. In order for implantation to occur and for there to be a pregnancy, the whole creative reproductive centre prepares for this process. The endometrium (the lining of the womb) is becoming thicker with nutrients ready to support new life. There is a build-up, or congestion, of energy in our creative centre, not only on the physical side but also on the emotional, mental and spiritual levels of our being to prepare for a pregnancy. If fertilization does not occur, then subconsciously we may see this as a missed opportunity.

Some may see the premenstrual phase as a last-ditch attempt to implant that creative seed, to get that project going, and as we are more open to our intuition we are able to see more clearly even what those desires are or what exactly is standing in our way. All this may lead to us feeling frustrated, angry and irritable! It may sound like a bit of an off-the-wall theory but, hey, it may make sense to some of you!

Treatments are discussed in more detail in Chapter 7, but you may find that making small changes to your diet and lifestyle may be all that is needed to help bring your smile back.

- *Diet*: eating sugary snacks may provide the initial comfort that you seek but the quick bursts of glucose may later give you headaches and make you feel hungry once again soon after reaching for that chocolate bar.
- *Caffeine*: whether coffee, chocolate, tea or soft drink, caffeine will make you more jittery and irritable.
- *Stress*: too much stress will worsen your mood and cause irritability.
- *Sleep problems*: if you're not getting enough sleep you may be more irritable and cranky during the day.

Anger

No one likes being angry! Some women may naturally have a mild-mannered disposition, whereas for others it may be entirely normal to exhibit heightened emotion. Wherever you fall in the 'angry spectrum', most women find that their level of aggression increases around the time of their periods. So are we just using our periods as a free licence to stomp around and exert our anger, or could there be a biological reason why we may become like this?

In biological terms fluctuations in behaviour following ovulation may occur with the purpose of promoting reproduction, in other words, with a view to becoming pregnant. Studies conducted in rats and other animals have shown that sexual receptivity increases and aggression decreases when oestrogen levels are high, just before ovulation. In the days following ovulation, if fertilization does not occur then oestrogen levels fall. This may lead to the opposite effect, of sexual receptivity decreasing and irritability increasing.

This basically means that once your ovary releases an egg, if you don't become pregnant then your period follows around 14 days later. During this time you may become irritable and less interested in sex, since (according to the theory) you've lost out on the incentive of falling pregnant.

Research has also shown that symptoms attributed to PMS tend to significantly reduce if not disappear altogether during times when our periods have temporarily been halted or cease altogether. As a result, instead of our sex hormone (oestrogen and progesterone) levels yoyo-ing up and down, they tend to be at a more constant level. This might happen, for example, during pregnancy, while taking certain types of contraceptives, and in women who have had their ovaries removed.

Short-term memory loss

There may be occasions around your period where you find that you are more forgetful than usual. It is often just short-term memory loss, where you're not able to recall where you put your car keys even though they were with you about five minutes ago! Although forgetfulness on its own may not be particularly distressing compared to other PMS-related symptoms, it should not be underestimated as it can lead to a feeling of insecurity, consequently providing the impetus for a lack of self-esteem.

So let's look at the scientific evidence! A recent study conducted in New York looked into the structural changes in the brain that occur during the menstrual cycle. Interestingly, they found that following menstruation, grey matter (the active part of the brain), was increased in the part of the brain that is responsible for short-term memory, the hippocampus. This suggests that our memory isn't so great just before and during our period, but reassuringly does seem to improve following our period.

Crying

Many women feel far more emotional than usual in the days leading up to their period. Some have found themselves bursting into tears for no apparent reason, while others simply feel more weepy than usual. You may have found that after cooking your partner his favourite meal he comments, 'That was lovely, dear, but perhaps a touch more salt next time.' You may not be able to see that this was merely a helpful suggestion as opposed to code language for 'I think we should split up!' During your period, your sex hormones are very up and down and so it's not surprising that you may feel a little off-centre.

In the previous sections we discussed the issue of depression in PMS and more specifically the role of serotonin. Just to recap quickly, scientific evidence strongly suggests a link between depression and having low levels of serotonin. Oestrogen helps raise serotonin levels via the action of MAO, whereas high levels of progesterone do the opposite and result in low mood. Since depression and low mood can be key features of PMS, it is not surprising that you may be more teary in order to help you deal with your internal feelings.

Interestingly, crying is not a simple process of the eyes going into tear overdrive, but a relatively complicated process. For a start, there are actually three different types of tears.

1 *Basal tears* are physiological tears, which aim to keep our eyes lubricated.
2 *Reflex tears* are produced in response to an irritant getting into our eyes, for example an eyelash, or the chemicals that are released when chopping onions.
3 *Emotional tears* are invariably produced following an emotional trigger such as watching a sad film.

The chemical components of tears vary depending on which one of the three types they are. Emotional tears have been shown to have higher levels of prolactin (a protein-based hormone), as well as leucine enkephalin (a natural painkiller). Some scientists have suggested that since there may be a link between levels of prolactin and depressive symptoms, the release of prolactin in tears is a way for the body to rid itself of prolactin and therefore reduce the levels of depression.

If you recall, the limbic system is the part of the brain responsible for mood, emotions and behaviour. The limbic system has also been shown to have control over the part of the nervous system that controls the tear glands and therefore it makes sense to say that when the limbic system is activated by a certain emotion it will in turn lead to the production of tears.

Experts believe that crying releases certain chemicals and hormones, which helps to explain the old maxim that everyone feels better after a good cry.

Insomnia

You find yourself in your most comfortable pair of pyjamas, your hot water bottle is at the ready and you're armed with your favourite blanket – but despite taking these measures you find that you're still having difficulty getting to sleep, or are waking up in the middle of the night because you're unable to get comfortable and generally feel restless.

Research has shown that women with severe forms of PMS perceive their quality of sleep to be poor in the premenstrual period. Studies have revealed conflicting results, with most concluding that there appears to be no direct link to illustrate particular alterations in the sleep pattern and PMS. According to the Edinburgh Sleep Centre, women are among the most chronically sleep-deprived members of society. This is thought to be due to a number of factors, for example responsibilities as a professional, homemaker and mother. The centre has also recognized that physiological differences resulting from fluctuations in hormones during the menstrual cycle add to the problem and has called this 'menstrual associated sleep disorder' (MASD). In MASD, sleep disturbance is most marked during the first two to three days of your period and although the exact mechanism is yet to be elucidated, it is thought to be something to do with falling progesterone levels leading to a reduction in rapid eye movement (REM) sleep. REM sleep is the stage of the sleep cycle when you are dreaming and the brain is most active.

Getting enough sleep is vitally important, as it gives your body the opportunity to recharge itself and prepare for the following day. Ideally, women should try to get seven hours of uninterrupted sleep every night in order to function to their full potential and enhance their overall quality of life. The Royal College of Psychiatrists has advised on some self-help tips to ensure you get as many of those forty winks as possible!

Here are some simple tips that many people have found helpful.

- Keep your bedroom as a sanctuary of rest – you need a place to subconsciously associate with sleep. Make sure that your bed and bedroom are comfortable – not too hot, not too cold, not too noisy.
- Make sure that your mattress supports you properly. It should not be so firm that your hips and shoulders are under pressure or so soft that your body sags. Generally, you should replace your mattress every ten years to get the best support and comfort.
- Get some exercise. Don't overdo it, but try some regular swimming or walking. The best time to exercise is in the daytime – particularly late afternoon or early evening. Exercising later than this may disturb your sleep.
- Try to avoid working or studying in your bedroom – it should be a place to wind down.
- Take some time to relax properly before going to bed. Some people find aromatherapy helpful.
- If something is troubling you, and there is nothing you can do about it right away, try writing it down before going to bed and then tell yourself to deal with it tomorrow.
- If you can't sleep, get up and do something you find relaxing. Read, watch television or listen to quiet music. After a while you should feel tired enough to go to bed again.

If you find that despite taking these measures you're still having problems sleeping then it would certainly be worth consulting your doctor. Although not conclusive, there is some evidence to suggest that starting the oral contraceptive pill may help regulate your sleep through the action of regulating your sex hormones.

Low energy

During your period and just before it you may find it an extra effort to do the household chores, to make it to this week's Pilates class or even stay up late to watch your favourite movie. You find that you're exhausted even though you really haven't taken on too many physical stresses. You may feel that you're lacking energy and this may be for a combination of reasons. As discussed earlier, you may find that your quality of sleep isn't as good; the fact that you're feeling low may mean that you're not in the mood to go out jogging this evening; you may be suffering with a headache and therefore would prefer to rest in order to let it pass.

There could be other reasons too. Cortisol is a hormone involved in the body's stress response. An excess of cortisol can cause anxiety and insomnia, whereas a deficiency can lead to depression and lethargy. One study found that women with PMS-related depression had an imbalance of cortisol levels, compared to women who had few or no PMS symptoms. Another study found that women with PMS-related depression had lower night-time cortisol levels than women without these symptoms.

You can boost your energy levels by trying simple measures. For example, incorporating complex carbohydrates into your diet, such as rice, bread and pasta, should avoid the glucose highs and lows that are associated with eating refined sugars such as sweets and chocolates. It should also ensure that your energy levels remain at a more constant level.

There are a number of vitamins that all work in slightly different ways with the ultimate goal being to boost energy levels. Try supplementing your diet with foods rich in the B vitamins and co-enzyme Q10, found in some types of fish and organ meats like liver and kidneys. If that doesn't whet your appetite then simply try taking the vitamin supplements available from chemists. However, do seek advice from your doctor before doing so.

Anxiety

Many women report feeling more anxious than usual in the days leading up to their period. They find that what would normally be perceived as a minor issue leaves them feeling 'on edge' and jittery.

Recently there has been much interest in a substance called 'allopregnanolone', which is basically a neuro-steroid – a type of hormone that's related to nerves in the brain. Allopregnanolone is a hormone produced by the adrenal gland, which sits just above your kidneys. The adrenal gland is also responsible for the production of other hormones such as adrenalin and noradrenalin (which explains their names). Allopregnanolone is normally released at times of stress. It exerts its effects by targeting certain 'GABA' receptors in the brain in order to reduce anxiety and create calm at times of stress.

Don't be too distracted by the medical names for now; the main point to understand is that scientists believe that this hormone may be responsible for anxiety and other mood disorders reported in PMS patients. Studies have shown that during the luteal phase of the menstrual cycle there are reduced levels of allopregnanolone. Since we now know that this hormone is responsible for inducing a state of calmness at times of stress, it could help to explain the occurrence of heightened anxiety levels that occur on a cyclical basis around your period.

Positive PMS symptoms

Although it may be difficult to convince you, PMS doesn't have to consist of a week full of doom, gloom and despair. Some women have reported experiencing positive PMS symptoms; and perhaps they are simply a proportion of the lucky few. While there's no denying that for some women PMS can be extremely distressing and debilitating, for others, however, changing your perception of PMS may prove beneficial. Some of the upsides to PMS include:

- it confirms you are not pregnant;
- it reminds you that your body is continuing to work as usual;
- the perception of having plumper, more attractive breasts;
- more energy than usual;
- more creative ideas;
- increased sexual interest and enjoyment;
- increased sexual desire.

Summary

- Depression – occurs due to low levels of serotonin in the brain; oestrogen increases it and progesterone decreases it.
- Irritability and aggression – following ovulation, oestrogen levels fall, which also reduces the levels of serotonin, leading to depressed mood and irritability.
- Anger – reduced levels of oestrogen may be linked to aggression.
- Short-term memory loss – the result of structural changes in the brain's memory centre, the hippocampus, during the menstrual cycle.
- Crying – due to low levels of serotonin. Crying is also a coping mechanism to help 'wash away' the problems.
- Sleep problems – physiological differences resulting from fluctuations in hormones during the menstrual cycle can lead to poor sleep.
- Low energy – thought to be due to an imbalance in cortisol levels, which is normally involved in the body's stress response.
- Anxiety – allopregnanolone normally during times of stress induces a state of calm. It is thought that low levels are released premenstrually, resulting in anxiety.
- Positive PMS symptoms – despite the vast array of physical and emotional discomforts that are synonymous with PMS, there are upsides too!

6

Physical symptoms

Just before and during the proverbial 'time of the month' most women tend not to feel 100 per cent themselves. Their symptoms can vary from mild headaches, bizarre food cravings and the thought of feeling unattractive, to full-on psychosis.

Approximately 5–8 per cent of women have the misfortune of experiencing symptoms at the far end of the spectrum whereby their behaviour is often irrational, volatile and can affect their ability to function normally. In 1987 premenstrual dysphoric disorder (PMDD) was described as a condition that encompasses the extreme symptoms, and it's obvious to say that this is no laughing matter for the women affected. Fortunately, most women fall somewhere in the middle of a vast spectrum of symptoms and may simply find that they're more sensitive, both physically and emotionally, than is normal for them.

During your premenstrual period, you may notice some people commenting that you are moody and even difficult to be around at times. One minute you may find that your insides feel like they're on fire and the next as if someone's thrown a bucket of cold water over you. You may find yourself being more sensitive to comments, especially those relating to your appearance, when on any other day you wouldn't normally give two hoots when someone comments that your red shoes don't quite match the colour of your lipstick or that your roots need re-highlighting! You may also notice that your clothes don't fit quite as comfortably as they did last week and you may be wearing your bra on a slightly looser notch.

We've already spoken about how the spectrum and severity of premenstrual symptoms can vary greatly between individuals. However, if you speak to your girlfriends about this you may find certain symptoms tend to be more common and experienced more frequently. Some of these may include bloating, breast tenderness or swelling, headaches, diarrhoea, abdominal cramps and cravings as well as many others.

So are these emotional and physical fluctuations simply an unfortunate injustice to womankind or could it be due to other reasons? Well, the simple answer is that premenstrual syndrome basically comes down to the actions of the sex hormones, oestrogen and progesterone, and the way they interact with various parts of your body, resulting in a multitude of symptoms.

Research has shown that symptoms attributed to PMS tend to significantly reduce, if not disappear altogether, during times when our periods have temporarily been halted or cease altogether. This seems to be related to the fact that instead of our sex hormone levels yoyo-ing up and down, they tend to be at a more constant level; for example, during pregnancy, when taking certain types of contraceptives and in those women who have had their ovaries removed.

During the course of this chapter we try and elucidate scientific reasons that may explain the symptoms associated with PMS. So let's explore some of the more common symptoms and try to seek out biological explanations, to prove that we're not making it up!

Bloating

Many women complain of a fullness in the tummy, feeling bloated or a general discomfort when wearing certain clothing just before or during their period. They may feel larger than usual and attribute this weight gain to 'water retention'. However, studies have so far shown no objective evidence for extra water being retained during this time, suggesting that it's a subjective 'feeling' rather than any actual bloating itself.

There are two possible theories to explain the sensation of tummy bloating: it may result from reduced tolerance to physical discomfort while in an altered mood state, or from changes in the response of certain tissues to hormones.

In support of the latter theory, one Norwegian study found that changes in the permeability (or leakiness) of tiny blood vessels (called capillaries) in the body resulted in the redistribution of body fluids during the luteal phase of the menstrual cycle. Blood vessels may therefore leak extra fluid into the tissues around the body, so that although there is no extra water in your body, it's more obvious because it's not just in the blood but in your tummy, or arms or legs.

Lots of women report gaining one or two pounds in weight during the lead-up to their period. This may simply be because certain food cravings premenstrually may result in binge-eating. Also, during your period headaches and lethargy may mean that you feel less inclined to exercise, so limited physical activity combined with increased appetite may lead to weight gain.

Despite what science tells us, some women find that they do benefit from taking natural diuretics such as asparagus, celery and dandelion. Simple measures such as having a cup of dandelion tea once in a while could help to lose water. Interestingly, treatment aimed at influencing brain activity, for example antidepressants, has been shown to improve discomfort related to bloating in some women, so that if you're in a better state of mind, chemicals in your brain may not perceive the sensation of bloating as so uncomfortable. It is thought that this is because the brain alters the way in which we perceive such symptoms.

Bloating may also make you feel lethargic and therefore less inclined to exercise. However, do try and get out in the open air every day: 30 minutes of gentle exercise may be all that is required to help improve matters, making you feel more alert and positive.

Breast tenderness

Many women report breast tenderness around the time of their period, and of those approximately 8–10 per cent experience moderate to severe breast pain. Breast discomfort that occurs just before your period and settles shortly after bleeding stops is most probably the result of hormonal fluctuations during your monthly cycle. The medical term used to describe this is 'cyclical mastalgia'. Mastalgia means pain in the breasts and as the name suggests this form of mastalgia occurs regularly on a cyclical basis, often until the menopause, and can interfere with day-to-day activities.

The anatomy of breast tissue varies quite significantly depending on where you are in your monthly cycle and is very sensitive to the effects of oestrogen and in particular progesterone. Approximately five to seven days following the end of your period, breast volume is at its lowest, which is thought to be due to a reduction in the levels of circulating progesterone. Progesterone levels peak just before the onset of your period and result in the accumulation of fluid around milk ducts, causing engorgement which leads to stretching of nerve fibres. This stretching results in the sensation of pain.

Another study suggests that the hormone prolactin may have a role to play in premenstrual breast tenderness. Prolactin is normally responsible for enlargement of the mammary glands (the milk-makers) in breast tissue and also milk production post-pregnancy. It is secreted by the brain in a pulsatile fashion even while not pregnant and it is thought that premenstrual breast pain is most likely due to a surge in prolactin levels. Some women release more than normal amounts of prolactin in response to stressful situations and during deep sleep phases, and this appears to stimulate the breast tissue and may cause breast pain.

It is important to remember that breast pain cannot always be attributed to PMS. There are other causes, such as fibrocystic breast disease, use of the pill, benign cysts, to name a few. It is certainly worth speaking to your doctor if you are in any way worried or find that your symptoms fail to settle on their own.

The best way to manage symptoms is to start by taking simple measures. Wearing a well-fitting supportive bra is often all that is needed to make a world of difference. Applying heat packs may help in relieving pain. Research has suggested that chasteberry, a fruit native to Mediterranean Europe and Central Asia, may help in the suppression of raised prolactin levels by blocking the part of the brain that is responsible for its release. This is discussed in more detail in Chapter 7.

Headaches

So far we've learned that in order for our menstrual cycle to run like clockwork, our sex hormones are cleverly at work in a complex but well-orchestrated sequence acting on the brain, ovaries and the womb. Oestrogen and progesterone have strong effects on certain areas in the brain which are responsible for our mood and the way we perceive pain. They also alter the lining of the womb (endometrium) and stimulate the production of other hormones and chemicals important for the normal functioning of the menstrual cycle. So why are we harping on about oestrogens again and what relevance do they have to those annoying headaches you may experience around the time of your period?

Well, although it's not entirely clear, it seems that altering levels of sex hormones, particularly oestrogen, appears to be related to headaches associated with PMS – 'menstrual migraines'. Research has shown that headaches related to PMS seem to involve the brain itself, as opposed to being the result of tension of the scalp muscles, which causes a different type of headache called a 'tension headache'. It has also been suggested that particular nerves in the brain that are involved in the 'pain-modulating system' through the action of serotonin may alter our perception of pain and our 'headache threshold'.

We already know that the normal female life cycle is associated with a number of hormonal milestones, such as:

- menarche – the very first period
- pregnancy
- use of the 'pill'
- the menopause – the cessation of periods
- the use of HRT – hormone replacement therapy.

It seems that all of these events result in alterations in sex hormone levels and may cause a change in the prevalence or intensity of headaches. In further support of this, many studies have suggested a link between headaches and migraines and the female sex hormones. Interestingly, twice as many women experience headaches as men, and attacks are most frequently noted from the onset of puberty, which further supports the role of hormones in their occurrence.

Research has found that hormone replacement with oestrogen can worsen migraines and oral contraceptives can change the character and frequency of migrainous headaches, suggesting that oestrogen levels in particular may be responsible for menstrually related headaches.

Generally different mechanisms can explain the headaches in

different women, but the key seems to be a change in hormone levels. Some women experience more frequent headaches once they become pregnant, or start taking the pill, while other women, for example those with menstrually related headaches, will have fewer headaches under the same conditions.

Diarrhoea and abdominal cramps

Many women find that their bowels are pretty haywire around the time of their period. An initial period of constipation is often quickly followed by diarrhoea. Some women may find that they need to visit the ladies' room more frequently than normal and for some venturing outdoors proves near impossible without knowing that there is a loo within a 50-yard radius of their whereabouts! So is it simply a nasty coincidence that your bowels have seemed temporarily to adopt a life of their own during the few days around your period, or can we be blame it on PMS again?

It seems that it's all down to the action of progesterone. Roughly about a week before starting your period, your progesterone levels are at their highest. Progesterone has the effect of making your bowels more relaxed and lazy by reducing the tone of the bowel wall and the mobility of smooth muscle. It therefore slows down gut activity, which may lead to constipation and a sensation of feeling bloated. During your period progesterone levels dramatically fall, which then produces the opposite effect, of diarrhoea and tummy cramps.

Tummy pains

Something that most of us have experienced at one time or another – yes, the female curse that we are only too familiar with, that is period pains! Just before the start of your period you're fast asleep only to be woken at some ungodly hour by the unbearable call of your uterus. It feels as if your womb is being used as a punch-bag for no justifiable reason. As if we didn't have enough to deal with, period pains are there to seal the premenstrual deal!

So let's take a look at why this happens. The medical term for painful periods is dysmenorrhoea, of which there are two types.

- *Primary dysmenorrhoea* describes the normal period pain experienced by many women around the time of their period where there is no underlying medical problem.
- *Secondary dysmenorrhoea* describes pain around the time of your period that's caused by an underlying problem, such as endometriosis or pelvic inflammatory disease. It is less common than primary dysmenorrhoea, and tends to affect women later in their reproductive lives.

We've already discussed the normal menstrual cycle in some detail in Chapter 3 and you may find it useful to refer back before reading on.

Period pains are essentially caused by the action of chemicals called prostaglandins. Prostaglandins are found in all tissues and organs including the womb, and serve a number of functions around the body. But the one we're most concerned with is their ability to constrict and dilate smooth muscle cells.

Ovulation occurs mid-cycle at around Day 14 for most women. There is a window of around three days following ovulation that allows fertilization to occur. In preparation for a potential pregnancy, progesterone levels rise, which results in the lining of the uterus becoming thicker. If fertilization does not occur, progesterone levels fall and the lining of the womb is shed as your monthly period. This bleeding is often accompanied by pain because in order to help the womb to expel the unwanted lining, prostaglandins act on the muscle cells in the wall of the uterus to cause it contract. It is these contractions of the uterus that lead to the sensation of tummy spasms.

Some women produce higher levels of prostaglandins, which may cause increased contractions of the uterus. These cramps may be more painful because there is reduced blood (and therefore oxygen) supply to the muscle wall of the uterus (myometrium) during the contractions. The pain is not always restricted to the tummy area; sometimes it can spread to the lower back and thighs. Unfortunately, around 15 per cent of women suffer with period pains that are severe enough to hamper daily activities.

There are a number of measures you can take to ensure that period pains cause as little disruption to your life as possible. If you're at home, simply placing a hot water bottle wrapped in a soft towel over your lower tummy may be all that is required to ease the pain.

Exercising may be the last thing you feel like doing during your period, but surprisingly you may find that you benefit from short bursts of gentle exercise like walking or cycling.

Having a nice hot soak in the bath with some muscle relaxants dissolved in the water may prove beneficial. Gentle massage over the painful area may also help.

If you find that despite trying these initial measures you are still having pain then there is a wide range of painkillers available over the counter that should help manage the pain.

Non-steroidal anti-inflammatory drugs (NSAIDs) work for approximately 70 per cent of women with period pains. They work by blocking the effects of prostaglandins (the main culprits in causing period pains). NSAIDs reduce the strength of the uterine contractions and subsequently reduce the discomfort that is caused. As their name suggests, NSAIDs also have additional actions that serve to reduce pain resulting from inflammation.

Ibuprofen and aspirin are part of the NSAID family of medications and can be purchased over the counter in most pharmacies. Pharmacists are a useful source of information – speak with them first to ensure that the medication is suitable for you. If you find that these medications are not helping your symptoms then it is worth visiting your GP, who may prescribe a stronger painkiller, such as mefanamic acid (another NSAID), and will examine you to ensure that there is no other reason for your pain.

If NSAIDs are either not suitable for you or you do not find them effective, alternative painkillers are available. Paracetamol, also easily available over the counter, has very few side-effects. However, studies have shown that paracetamol is not as effective in reducing pain compared to an NSAID.

If you need contraception as well as relief from period pain, your GP may discuss the role of the combined contraceptive pill (COCP) which may function as a way of alleviating pain as well as a contraceptive if needed. In terms of easing pain, the pill works in two ways: it thins the lining of the womb, and it helps to reduce the amount of prostaglandins that are released.

Types of contraceptive pill are discussed in Chapter 7.

Intolerance to heat

It's the middle of winter, you have the window open, you've already turned over your pillow to the cold side twice *and* you've thrown your quilt off the bed! So why is it that you're *still* feeling hot when the rest of the world is snugly tucked up under a warm duvet and has the heating turned up to maximum? Why are you tossing and turning and finding yourself unable to get comfortable no matter what you try?

Following ovulation (roughly about two weeks before your period is due), you have a slight rise in core body temperature which is caused by the increasing levels of progesterone and a substance called 3-alpha-pregnanolone which is produced when progesterone is metabolized and broken down.

This rise in body temperature is a very useful indicator for couples trying to conceive. They may have been advised to track the body temperature of the female partner in a diary form. Assuming the woman is fertile, she should find that a rise of 0.4 degrees Fahrenheit from her baseline temperature would indicate that ovulation has occurred, corresponding to the rising levels of progesterone. If you check your body temperature at the same time every day throughout your cycle this increase should be noticeable for about 48 hours after ovulation.

Cravings

Some women notice that they experience certain food cravings around the time of their period. These could be for anything but tend to involve 'feel-good' foods like crisps and chocolate – foods that are carbohydrate rich. So what's the story? Again, like everything else we've discussed so far, it's all to do with changes in hormone levels. This time it's to do with their effect on the brain through serotonin, one of the most important 'happy' hormones. Serotonin is a neurotransmitter, a chemical link between brain cells in various areas of the brain, allowing them to communicate with each other. It plays an important role in the modulation of appetite, as well as anger and mood which were discussed in greater detail in the previous chapter.

Serotonin levels are altered by different types of food and since serotonin is also linked to mood, the type of food you eat can have quite a significant impact on how you feel once you've eaten it. Food cravings can be the result of low serotonin levels in the brain; eating foods with a high carbohydrate content serves to raise the levels of serotonin and so improve your mood. Interestingly, one study found a staggering 61 per cent increase in energy intake during the premenstrual period! It is thought that the changes in energy intake parallel changes in your metabolism which are also dependent on menstrual changes in hormone levels.

Unfortunately, eating sugary and salty snacks in an erratic manner simply to get your 'fix' of serotonin is not a solution to end the cravings. The result is a quick upswing in your blood-sugar levels, followed by a rapid decline, which leaves you feeling hungry again. So what can we do to stifle that uncontrollable urge to visit the fridge at 3 a.m. for our third helping of chocolate mousse?

The best way to curb PMS cravings is to alter your eating *habits* in addition to *what* you eat. The British Dietetic Association (BDA) suggests an approach that aims to maximize serotonin production and therefore give a sense of satiety. An overall healthy diet based on lower fat and sugar intake, choosing more unrefined carbohydrate foods and including fruit and vegetables in good amounts is recommended.

Eating regular meals and snacks containing starchy carbs is a good way to prevent the peaks and troughs in blood-sugar levels. Avoid leaving longer than three hours without something to eat – just a piece of fruit is a healthy alternative to chocolate and biscuits and is often sufficient between meals to top up the blood sugar levels slowly and prevent you from getting too hungry between meals.

Aches and pains

You've probably heard of endorphins, also known as 'feel-good' hormones. They resemble the opiates in their ability to produce pain relief! Endorphins are released during strenuous exercise, excitement, and climax, and are the body's natural painkillers, promoting a sense of well-being.

One study looking at sensitivity to pain in women with premenstrual dysphoric disorder (PMDD, a severe form of PMS discussed in detail in Chapter 8) found that those affected displayed lower endorphin levels throughout the menstrual cycle and exhibited shorter pain threshold and tolerance times. It may be that low endorphins are a cause for these general aches and pains, which is good news as it means that they may be relieved by boosting your endorphins. Try some intense exercise or an adrenaline-rush sport – or sexual activity; not only will your partner appreciate it but you'll feel great too!

Joint laxity

There is little information available on the cause of this, but some women report aches around the joints and possible increasing laxity of the joints. As discussed in Chapter 3, the premenstrual reduction in oestrogen levels may loosen collagen protein fibres, so it's possible that it causes some premenstrual joint loosening and pains. This is as yet not well investigated.

Sensory function

As twenty-first-century women, we can rely on verbal communication, body language, letters, emails, SMS and so on, to get our point across and generally function in the world. Several millennia ago, however, our ancestors were less fortunate and had to make do with visual stimuli and their sense of sound and smell.

You have probably not even noticed that your ability to hear, see, smell and taste may vary throughout your cycle. Studies have shown that oestrogen can have a positive effect on hearing, with the auditory threshold being lowest, meaning your ability to hear being sharpest, around the time of ovulation. In contrast, your ability to hear is at its lowest during your period, when oestrogen levels are lower. Studies have also shown that your ability to smell and your visual acuity follow a similar pattern – they both improve during ovulation and subsequently decline around the time of your period.

But why? Well, it's thought that it's all to do with that old cliché of finding a mate. It's believed that females had to be on top form during their ovulation period in order to successfully secure a mate. That meant that to capture the proverbial Mr Right (albeit the Neanderthal version!), women were reliant on sensory cues both to appear more attractive and to be attracted.

Problem skin

And we thought problem skin was something that only affected teenagers! How disappointing is must be, therefore, to continue to get spots once you're well into your twenties. Acne is a common skin complaint that many people have been affected by to varying degrees at some stage of their lives. If you already have acne then you may have noticed that it worsens premenstrually. On the other hand, if your skin is relatively well behaved you may have noticed a tendency to break out just before your period is due. Premenstrual acne occurs in 44 per cent of women in the late luteal phase of the cycle, and a recent study showed that the incidence of premenstrual acne per menstrual period in these individuals was 63 per cent.

So, is there officially such a thing as premenstrual acne, and why does it occur? Let's start by discussing why acne occurs. Acne occurs due to the stimulation of sebaceous (oil-making) glands by testosterone, one of a group of hormones collectively known as androgens. While androgens are commonly thought of as 'male' hormones they are also produced by women, in much smaller quantities. Androgens stimulate the sebaceous glands and hair follicles in the skin and are most often the cause of hormone-related acne. Sometimes sebaceous glands become clogged by excess oil and dead skin cells. This may lead to bacteria invading the pores, resulting in inflammation giving the appearance of red and angry-looking pimples.

When sebaceous glands are overstimulated, around the time of menstruation, women of all ages tend to have flare-ups. Studies have shown that the sebaceous duct openings on the skin tend to be smallest during Days 15–20 of the cycle, increasing on Days 21–26 and then decreasing again in the two days before menstruation. Premenstrual acne on average was found to be the worst on Day 22.

Although not properly understood, it is also thought that oestrogen plays a role in the regulation of sebum production. Therefore, before your period, when oestrogen levels fall, sebum production is increased.

Summary

- Bloating – research suggests that it's a subjective feeling rather than due to 'water retention'. Exercise and natural diuretics such as asparagus, celery and dandelion may help.
- Breast tenderness – rising progesterone levels just before the onset of your period result in the accumulation of fluid around milk ducts causing engorgement, which leads to stretching of nerve fibres. This stretching results in the sensation of pain. Try to ease the pain by wearing a well-fitting supportive bra or heat packs placed over your breasts for a short time.
- Headaches – different mechanisms can explain the headaches in different women, but the key seems to be a change in hormone levels.
- Diarrhoea and abdominal cramps – progesterone makes your bowels more relaxed and lazy by reducing the tone of the bowel wall and the mobility of smooth muscle. This slows down gut activity, which may lead to constipation and a sensation of feeling bloated. During your period progesterone levels dramatically fall, which then produces the opposite effect, of diarrhoea and tummy cramps.
- Tummy pains – prostaglandins act on the muscle cells in the wall of the uterus causing it to contract during your period. It is these contractions of the uterus that lead to the sensation of tummy spasms.
- Heat intolerance – following ovulation there is a slight rise in core body temperature, caused by the increasing levels of progesterone and 3-alpha-pregnanolone which is produced when progesterone is metabolized and broken down.
- Cravings – serotonin levels are altered by different types of food. Since serotonin is linked to mood, the type of food you eat can have quite a significant impact on how you feel once you've eaten it.
- Aches and pains – most likely due to low endorphin levels, which can be boosted by physical and sexual activity.

- Joint laxity – not very well understood but thought to be due to the effect of reducing oestrogen, causing loosening of collagen protein fibres.
- Effects on sensory function – your sense of sound, smell, vision, and taste have all been shown to increase during ovulation and reduce premenstrually.
- Problem skin – due to an imbalance of androgen production and the reduction in oestrogen levels premenstrually.

7

Therapies

Introduction – different treatments

Premenstrual syndrome covers a huge spectrum of symptoms and severity – over 150 symptoms have been reported. Up to 80 per cent of women suffer to some degree, and while some find that their symptoms do not impinge much on their lives, others may find life intolerable because of the severity of their physical, mental or emotional distress in the days prior to their period. It is important to realize that there is no such thing as a lost cause, and while you may feel you've tried everything and nothing works, there are literally hundreds of therapies and approaches out there that work wonders for different symptoms, and different women.

In the search for a cure there are three key points to remember. First, you're an individual, and so is the way you experience PMS. Therefore an individual approach is needed for each woman. Aromatherapy might be a life-saver for one woman, while another may need medical hormone treatment. Your best friend may not be bothered in the slightest by her monthly bloating, accepting that it's a normal part of her cycle, whereas you may suffer with severe abdominal cramps, and therefore need help.

Second, it's easy to get disheartened if you can't find a cure, which may sometimes take a while. Don't give up. You may not have had much success with one approach, or even several, but there is still a wealth of options out there.

Third, there is a lot of rubbish, marketed as wonder-cures, but actually having very little or no benefit, and even potentially causing harm. In the midst of all this it's easy to wonder where to start or turn to next. We focus here on those approaches that have been formally investigated by the Royal College of Obstetricians and Gynaecologists (RCOG), and are included in their guidelines on managing PMS, published in December 2007.

These guidelines are not exhaustive but they do look critically at the treatments available, the evidence for them, and suggest a basic approach for every woman. As any newly qualified doctor will tell you, a systematic approach is crucial in treating any illness or set of symptoms. So first we look at the lifestyle or 'conservative' changes you can make; second, at the spectrum of current medical treatments, and third, at the alternative therapies available. We focus on how and why these might each make a difference, the evidence for them, and the best way to approach each.

At the end of the chapter is a summary of symptoms and the best way to treat them, listing conservative, medical and alternative suggestions for each group of symptoms. Chapter 8 specifically addresses those whose symptoms aren't helped by these measures and seem to be relentless or disabling.

Conservative – lifestyle changes

All women suffering with PMS can try to adopt certain lifestyle changes, which in themselves may be enough to improve symptoms. Being overweight is statistically a risk factor for PMS, so if you think you might be able to reduce your weight, ideally by sensible healthy eating and exercise, it is likely to help with your symptoms.

Look out for number one

Easier said than done in today's world of 'busy, busy, busy', but coping with PMS requires positive action and you need to invest a little in yourself. The lifestyle changes recommended for PMS can be incorporated into a busy schedule, but if you have a busy family or work life it's often all too easy to struggle on, hoping you'll get better but not having time to do much to help yourself. Although it may sound selfish, in the long run looking out for yourself and taking the time out that you need will help not only you but also those around you. You'll be much more use to them if you feel better and more relaxed.

In the premenstrual time everything seems harder and more difficult to cope with – physical symptoms, irritating neighbours, even the daily traffic on your way to work. It's crucial that you recognize and maybe even expect this, so that you can plan time for yourself to enable you to cope rather than just survive. You may need to make sure that your diary is free that week so that you can get a little more sleep, and perhaps plan some exercise or relaxation techniques. Even planning a hot bath and leaving the phone off the hook for a few hours may make a big difference. Of course, you need to think about your family and friends or those who depend on you, but ultimately PMS is just like anything else – you can't cope with it if you don't make time and give yourself the chance.

So if you haven't done so before, take the time to think about how you could adopt some of the following lifestyle changes to help improve your PMS symptoms, and also the way you yourself cope with them. Be realistic. You won't suddenly switch from running round madly all day every day, grabbing quick snacks, smoking, comfort eating and never exercising, to being a chilled-out organic food junkie who calms the storm wherever she goes. Initially, small changes are better than big ones if it means they're sustainable, and you need to find what works best for you.

Exercise

Although there aren't many scientific trials, it is widely agreed that exercise is beneficial in improving symptoms, as well as physical and emotional well-being. Many women report significant improvements with various different types of exercise. Exercise should always be balanced, with at least some aerobic compo-nent (to push your heart rate up and get you sweating). General health recommendations would be that you do at least 30 minutes of aerobic exercise three to four times a week. Aerobic exercise increases blood-flow to your brain and muscles, generates serotonin (the 'feel-good' hormone) and helps to relieve stress.

It's important to choose a type of exercise that you enjoy and see it as time out for yourself to de-stress, making you feel healthier and happier with your body. Swimming, running and gym classes, and even walking for pleasure are all great examples. You may want to take up a dancing class with a friend or start brisk evening walks with a neighbour or partner after work. If the thought does not inspire you, try to be imaginative. Belly-dancing classes, pole dancing and line dancing are all potentially crazy-sounding but good fun and great exercise, with the added benefit of potentially involving a lot of laughter – which we all know is the very best medicine.

Exercise is often put on the back-burner as something we all know we should do more of but never have time for, so make a point to put it in your diary just as you would a meeting or coffee with a friend. If you don't currently exercise set small, short-term targets, for example, 'I will try three or four different exercise sessions in the next month. I can then decide which I prefer and spend the following month incorporating it into my schedule.'

Being on your feet all day at work, lugging the kids around or lifting boxes around the house may be very hard work, making you sweat and pushing your heart rate up, but they are not the kind of exercise we're talking about. While it's good that you're active, part of the value of exercise is finding something you enjoy; exercise should be for your benefit and not just another stressful, tiring part of your daily activities. Therefore you should find a type of exercise that you enjoy, and take time out to do it.

Other types of exercise, such as yoga, Pilates or martial arts, which focus as much on relaxation as the physical activity component, have been reported by some women to be tremendously effective. They give you time to relax and focus on something other than your stressful environment, as well as toning and benefiting the body itself. We would suggest that if you decide to take up an activity like this you join a class or hire an instructor to get the maximum benefit. DVDs may be helpful further down the line if you want to try it at home, but you may risk injuring yourself by not doing the moves correctly, and also you will not be escaping the stresses at home that are part of the problem (imagine trying to 'surrender to the stretch' of a yoga video with your kids fighting in the next room).

Whatever exercise you decide to do make sure it's enjoyable, achievable, and ideally done with a friend, so that you can encourage each other to keep on with it on days when it's raining or you feel tired – it really will make you feel better.

Diet

The dietary changes advised for helping with PMS are not that different from general healthy eating advice. Although again the evidence is not very robust, it is generally believed that lots of saturated fats and highly refined carbohydrates are not good for you – regardless of your PMS, they will make your mood worse and less predictable.

Too much alcohol and caffeine can dehydrate you, also playing havoc with your body's ability to moderate your mood; it is therefore likely to make you irritable and depressed, as well as depriving you of the refreshing sleep you need most. Ideally you should keep your alcohol intake well below the recommended maximum of 14 units a week (with no more than three to four units in one day). It has been suggested that caffeine intake should be below 400 mg in a day, which equates to about four cups of coffee or eight average cups of tea. In practice this may be a lot more than is helpful, and you may find that reducing your caffeine intake to a minimum, and having none after mid-afternoon, makes a big difference to your sleep and general well-being.

For a basic healthy diet, the Food Standards Agency recommends that your meals should be based around starchy foods, with about a third of what you eat being carbohydrates, a third being fruit and vegetables and a third made up of the other food groups – meat, fish, dairy products and everything else. The British Dietetic Association also provides good practical advice on healthy eating, including how to eat to improve your mood.

Aim to include the following in your diet, in balance:

- *Complex carbohydrates* (such as granary or wholemeal bread, brown rice, and bulgar wheat). These enable your body to have a slower energy release, and help prevent the energy highs and lows that can make your mood swings worse. The general idea is that the less refined and processed the carbohydrate is, the more nutrients are left in it (including fibre) and also the longer it will take for your body to break it down in the gut. Aim for products with a low glycaemic index (GI). The lower the GI, the more complex the carbohydrate and the less likely it is to cause a sudden surge in blood-sugar levels. Don't get caught out – wholemeal granary bread with lots of grains is best and often has a lower GI than plain brown bread. Brown bread can actually be quite refined, having had some of the bran removed from the wheat; it may even contain food colouring to make it look brown and healthier.

- *A good variety and amount of fruit and vegetables.* Five portions of fruit and vegetables a day should be a minimum, and should include as many different varieties as possible. Five different fruits or vegetables are much better for you than six of the same thing. Cabbage, watercress, okra, and dried figs in particular contain relatively high levels of calcium, which is believed to help prevent PMS and reduce symptoms. (This is discussed further below, in the section on alternative therapies and supplements.) Green, leafy vegetables contain magnesium; if your magnesium levels are low this could be exacerbating your PMS – so aspiring to follow in Popeye's footsteps may not be the only reason to eat your spinach. Antioxidants, widely publicized because of their ability to mop up harmful chemicals in the body, are much more effective when you get them from a variety of fruit and veg in your diet rather than supplements.
- *Plenty of fibre.* It has been suggested that fibre helps your body to get rid of excess oestrogen, although whether this actually affects PMS symptoms is unknown. It should, however, certainly help reduce the constipation and bloating that many women experience as part of their PMS. While some women may be over-zealous in their fibre intake, resulting in diarrhoea and possibly excess gas and wind, the majority of women have much less fibre in the diet than the recommended 20–35 g a day. A variety of types of fibre is important – getting all your fibre from one source (such as high-bran breakfast cereals) can cause increased bloating and gas. Choose a balance of high-fibre foods including oats, fresh and dried fruit and vegetables, and wholegrain products such as rice, pasta and cereals.
- *Protein* (from a variety of sources – meat, fish, seeds and nuts). This is not only necessary for bodily functions like growth and repair; it will also help you to feel full after your meals. Be aware that too much protein can actually be detrimental; aim to have about 35–45 g a day. A roasted chicken breast contains

about 27 g of protein; a small tin of tuna or a cod fillet contains about 24 g.

- *Plenty of water.* Try to drink at least 6 8 glasses a day. There is no evidence that bottled water is any better for you than tap water, unless you prefer the taste or it prompts you to drink more. If you suffer from premenstrual headaches these are almost certainly going to be worse if you are dehydrated. If you suffer from migraines these may be prolonged if you are dehydrated when a migraine starts.

- *'Good' fat.* Too much fat is definitely bad for you, contributing to problems with weight gain and general poor health. However, your body does need a certain amount of fat, so only ever having low-fat foods is not good either. The average woman should consume approximately 70 g of fat per day. Saturated fats, found in animal and dairy products should be kept to a minimum. So also should foods high in trans fats, or partially hydrogenated vegetable oils. These fats are made from vegetable oil that is chemically altered to make it turn solid, and are commonly found in foods like biscuits and pastry. Both of these types of fats contribute to heart disease and unhealthy weight gain, and should be replaced by a combination of unsaturated fats (mainly found in seeds and nuts) and omega-3 fatty acids (found particularly in oily fish such as salmon and mackerel). It can be difficult to suddenly switch your diet, but you could try having seeds and nuts to snack on at work one day a week, and maybe try a 'Fish Friday' once in a while.

It has been suggested that various foods may make your PMS worse. These include dairy and wheat products. There is actually little evidence from any research that these contribute to PMS in the general population, but some women have found that cutting them out of the diet helps. We would advise against food 'fads' and fanaticism, but if you feel this may help, the best idea is to exclude whatever you feel is contributing to your PMS from your diet. Avoid it for about three months (be militant about it!), and see if you notice a difference. Then consider reintroducing the food to see whether symptoms return. There is no point in avoiding a food or food group for the rest of your life if something totally unrelated has actually eased your symptoms. If reintroducing it brings back your symptoms again, then totally avoid the relevant food.

Bloating and water retention are likely to be worsened by high salt intake so try to avoid crisps and processed foods. Put black pepper or herbs rather than salt on your food to flavour it. You shouldn't have more than 6 g of salt a day. The majority of our salt intake usually comes from processed foods, which may even be marked as healthy (such as low-fat sauces or cereals) but are high in salt to enhance their flavour. On food labels the sodium content is often listed; remember that the salt content is actually two and a half times the sodium content.

It has been suggested that vitamin B6 (pyridoxine) eases PMS. It has been investigated quite extensively, with trials involving nearly 1,000 women, and the evidence for supplements at a low enough dose to be safe is not very convincing. However, ensuring that you have enough in your diet is probably a good idea. You need about 1.2 mg a day and you should be able to get enough from your diet, although you may want to try boosting your levels without taking supplements. Vitamin B6 is water-soluble and cannot be stored in the body. It is found in a wide variety of foods, including oats, rice, eggs, chicken, pork and potatoes. The best sources are probably fortified cereals and baked potatoes (with the skin still on). You could consider including spreads like Bovril or Marmite in your diet which contain added B vitamins – in moderation, of course! A level of no more than 10 mg a day is recommended as vitamin B6 can have toxic effects in high doses, but this is unlikely if your B6 just comes from your diet.

On a positive note, eating regularly, ideally every three hours, is recommended by many health specialists to keep your blood-sugar levels constant. This can be a small meal or a banana, but it is best not to go without food for too long as you are more likely to over-indulge if you're really hungry. This will result in a big rise in your blood-sugar level, and then a rebound dip which will make you feel rubbish. Again, aim to have foods with a low or medium GI to keep the release of energy into your bloodstream constant.

Katharina Dalton, one of the pioneers into research and under-standing of PMS, suggests a three-hour starch diet based on the idea of keeping your blood sugars stable by eating the right foods regularly throughout the day. You may find it helpful to explore this if you find you are prone to mood swings and think you might have soaring and plummeting blood sugars.

Many women are anaemic (have a low level of haemoglobin in the blood) as a result of heavy periods or poor dietary intake of iron. This makes it harder for blood to carry enough oxygen around the body, leading to tiredness and weakness. Being anaemic is certainly likely to make premenstrual tiredness, palpitations and abdominal cramps worse. If you suffer from heavy periods or think you may be anaemic it's worth seeing your GP to discuss this. They may do a blood test to check whether your blood count is low.

Iron supplements are sometimes necessary, but not very nice to take as they can cause constipation and bloating, so it's best to make sure you have plenty of iron in your diet to prevent anaemia. Spinach, broccoli and red meat are all great sources. Also important to remember is that your body's ability to absorb this iron is increased by vitamin C and decreased by tannins in tea and red wine. So if you take an iron supplement, have it with a glass of orange juice – not your morning cup of tea!

The hardest dietary aspect of PMS for a lot of women is the insatiable craving for sweet foods, especially chocolate. You may be able at least to reduce these by practical measures such as deliberately not having any in the house to tempt you, eating regular small, healthy meals to keep your blood sugar stable and eating foods containing the magnesium that some people believe your body is craving from the chocolate (such as almonds, cashew nuts, artichokes, spinach). Most importantly, remember that you are only human; abstinence is likely to result in binges, and a little treat once in a while is wise as well as kind. If you decide to indulge, buy small bars, try not to accept boxes of chocolates as gifts, and if possible buy dark rather than milk or white. And don't beat yourself up when you slip up – you're the only one to suffer for it after all.

Lastly, saffron has recently been suggested to be of benefit for PMS, with small studies showing it to reduce PMS symptoms, including depression, significantly more than a placebo. The amounts used were small (30 mg a day) and the study didn't look at dietary intake, but there may be some benefit from including it in the diet. As an example, when considering how to include your recommended weekly portions of oily fish in your diet, you could try experimenting with a healthy home-made paella, laden with saffron, to boost your mood in the week before you come on. Or what about a 'saffron party', with friends bringing different foods containing saffron? It may or may not help with your PMS, but could be a fun experiment!

Stress

Whether stress makes your PMS worse or makes you less able to deal with your symptoms, reducing your stress levels is likely to significantly improve how you feel each month. Easier said than done, I hear you say, but it is easy to get into such negative thinking that you give in to those things that you could in fact change, making life much more bearable.

For example, some things can't be changed. You may have young children that need constant attention, feeding, getting ready for school, and such like. But is there anyone who could feed them for you once in a while – a grandparent, a neighbour or friend with children nearby, to give you the chance to go to the gym or have a long bath to yourself? You may find every morning so stressful getting them ready for school that your day seems doomed from the start. Ask your partner to give you a hand a couple of days a month when you're struggling. Talk to your boss about working late a couple of days at the beginning of your cycle so you can start later when you know you're going to be feeling worse premenstrually.

Sit down and make a list of those things that make you feel stressed or not in control of your life. Then list what you can do to reduce them, especially before your period. Now set targets for when you will do some of these things. One of the main causes of stress is feeling that you're not in control, so focus on how you can regain a sense of control over your individual circumstances.

Sharing your stresses will also help to reduce them. Moaning on and on about the same problem may not be productive, but talking things through with a friend or partner, and planning together how to reduce your stress levels or help each other out can make a big difference. If you genuinely feel there is no one you can talk to, see your GP to arrange a few sessions with a counsellor, or join a local PMS support group. A problem shared can help you put it into perspective – and maybe even halve it.

Relaxation techniques have been shown to have some effect on improving depression and stress that is not related to PMS. Although not as good as antidepressants or cognitive behavioural therapy (discussed in Chapter 8) they may help improve low mood, and therefore could potentially be helpful for stress or feeling low due to PMS. There have been very limited, small and poorly conducted trials assessing the effect of recognized relaxation techniques on women's experience of PMS, which means the evidence for such techniques is scant. Relaxation techniques are therefore not routinely recommended, but since they seem to be effective for other conditions, and are easy to do if you suffer from premenstrual stress, anxiety or depression you may want to try them. There are various types of relaxation techniques which generally involve lying or sitting in a comfortable, neutral position and taking about 15 minutes to focus on gradually relaxing each part of the body individually.

Medical treatments

If your symptoms are not relieved by any of the lifestyle changes mentioned above, or you feel that they are severe enough to be affecting your life and you need help *now*, you should talk to your GP.

Many women complain that their GP doesn't have time for them or won't listen. Of course, in an ideal world all GPs would be attentive listeners with time to devote to everyone. Sadly this isn't always the case, however; if possible book a double appointment to give you time to sit down properly and discuss your concerns. If your GP is difficult to talk to, doesn't believe you, or tries to fob you off, try a different one. There's nothing wrong with asking friends or colleagues to find a GP who appears to be genuinely considerate and helpful. Ask your practice whether they have a doctor with a special interest in women's health. Giving up on conventional medicine because of one unhelpful GP is not necessarily the best move, especially if your PMS is adversely affecting your life.

A lot of the medical therapy for PMS is for those with more severe symptoms, and therefore discussed in Chapter 8.

Hormone therapy

In the past the oral contraceptive pill has been used to treat PMS by GPs but it has not always been effective, possibly because of the man-made type of progesterone (progestogen) in it. The pill comes in essentially two forms. One is progestogen only; the other is a combined pill, containing oestrogen and progestogen. Progestogen as a therapy on its own is discussed below; the type of pill we're talking about here is the combined oral contraceptive pill (COCP).

Theoretically, giving the pill stops your body from producing its own hormone cycle, as it is 'tricked' by these extra hormones into acting as though you were pregnant. You therefore don't ovulate, and the monthly hormonal changes are much reduced. Unfortunately, the progestogen in the pill is man-made, so is not quite the same as your body's own progesterone. The older types of pill contain a particular type of man-made progestogen with a similar structure to certain steroid hormones that can cause things like acne, weight gain, irritability and fluid retention. For this reason, these pills do not always help with PMS, as you are stopping your own troublesome hormone cycle, but replacing it with another troublesome hormone. Fortunately, in the last few years a new type of man-made progestogen has been developed, which is much less like the steroid hormones, and much kinder on your body in terms of side effects.

This type of progesterone, known as drospirenone, is found in a pill called Yasmin. A new, lower dose of this pill, Yaz, is currently available in the USA and has been shown to be effective for PMS. There are other pills containing similar types of newer progesterone, made by different manufacturers; examples of these are Mercilon, Femodette and Minulet.

Some of these pills are associated with a slightly higher risk of developing blood clots in the legs (deep vein thrombosis) and lungs (pulmonary embolism); your doctor should check that you don't have any risk factors for these conditions before giving you the pill. To put this risk-taking into perspective, if you are not on the pill or pregnant your risk of a potentially dangerous blood clot is 5 in 100,000. If you take an older version of the pill for a year this risk grows to 15 in 100,000. With some of the newer pills this risk goes up to about 25 in 100,000 – still a tiny risk but significantly higher. Some women cannot take the pill for other medical reasons; if you want to try it or have any concerns you should discuss them with your GP.

Progesterone

Progesterone is the hormone released by the body during the menstrual cycle and belongs to a group of hormones known as progestogens. The term progestogen is also used to refer to man-made hormones that are very similar to natural progesterone.

It has been suggested that PMS might be caused by low levels of progesterone, and therefore that it might be a good treatment. Progesterone is often given in different forms for contraception, for example the progesterone-only pill, or the depot progestogen injection. This is a contraceptive injection that slowly releases synthetic progesterone into the body over several months to provide contraception, in a similar way to the progesterone-only pill, but by a single injection every few months instead of daily tablets. Unfortunately a number of the symptoms of PMS are also side effects of these contraceptives. Hence giving depot progestogen injection might reduce premenstrual symptoms, but actually make you experience constantly slightly reduced versions of these same symptoms for the following three months – not so good!

A number of clinical trials have looked at the effectiveness of giving progesterone or progestogens for PMS, compared with a placebo. Progesterone can be given in tablet form or vaginally, but there is very little evidence that either is any more effective than a placebo. In the past it has been advocated as a treatment, but with minimal scientific evidence to back it up. One trial showed a significant benefit from rectal and vaginal pessaries of natural progesterone, but several other trials showed no effect.

If either is to be used, natural progesterone rather than progestogen is likely to be the most effective, and best applied as a cream or suppository rather than taken as a tablet. It could be considered in severe PMS, but there is currently very little evidence for it, and it is therefore not recommended as standard treatment.

Other medical treatments

Your doctor might suggest or prescribe other medications to help with the symptoms rather than the root cause of your PMS. For example, they might advise regular ibuprofen to help with headaches or abdominal pains. This not only helps with pain, but may also act on the muscle in the womb itself to help reduce cramping effects.

Another medication that used to be more widely used for PMS is the diuretic, commonly known as a 'water pill'. This type of medication increases the amount of water that the kidneys flush out from the body, and therefore helps to reduce water retention, particularly in high blood pressure. In the past this has been prescribed for the bloating and possible water retention associated with PMS. However, it is not shown to have much effect on reducing bloating. In fact it could make you dehydrated as your body is forced to get rid of more water than it really wants to; it is therefore not recommended. If you feel that you suffer from premenstrual water retention, particularly around the legs and ankles, you should see your doctor for a full discussion of the risks and benefits of diuretics before you start taking them.

Natural diuretics, such as dandelion extract, nettle leaf and cider vinegar are often marketed for premenstrual abdominal bloating and fluid retention. The effectiveness of these has not been well investigated, and there is a lack of objective evidence that they improve symptoms compared with a placebo. If stronger, medically proven diuretics (which remove water from the body to the extent that they could leave you dehydrated) do not improve bloating it's probably unlikely that natural diuretics will have a better effect. However, some women report beneficial effects and because of the lack of evidence either way it's difficult to be sure. We would suggest you see a doctor before using diuretics of any kind because of the potential problems they could have and also to rule out any other cause of bloating or leg swelling.

Alternative therapies

There are two main concerns that conventional medics have about alternative therapies. First there is the lack of scientific evidence for their effectiveness. This does not mean that they don't work, but that we don't know whether they work or not. Second, if they have not been scientifically studied we don't know whether or not they are safe. 'Natural' obviously doesn't necessarily mean 'safe' – there are plenty of poisonous plants around that without too much preparation could easily have a number of very unpleasant effects on you, making you vomit horribly, or even stopping your heart. Because they are not regulated, different preparations of the same extract may have very different concentrations, so one may potentially be safe and another may not. Equally, there are lots of remedies that have been used for hundreds of years, been found time and again to be very safe and effective, and have just not been investigated in large 'scientific' trials, and consequently are not medically recommended. It is therefore important when venturing into alternative medicine for the first time to be aware of these issues, to be informed, to find a practitioner that you can trust, and aim to keep an open mind.

Herbal extracts/supplements

The best evidence for any alternative therapies or supplements is for agnus castus, calcium and/or vitamin D, and magnesium supplements.

Agnus castus

Vitex agnus castus, or vitex or chasteberry, is a plant naturally found around the Mediterranean, Africa and Central Asia. Its leaves, berries and flowers can all be harvested to produce extracts for medicinal purposes. Chemicals quite similar to hormones in the body have been extracted from the plant, and it may be these that cause its effect; or it may be related to how it helps modify the body's response to stress.

Doses of 20 mg a day have been shown to be significantly more effective than a placebo at reducing anger, irritability, mood disturbances, headaches and breast tenderness associated with PMS. It is believed to be safe, with only mild, reversible side effects reported.

The RCOG recognizes it as one of the most effective alternative treatments for PMS, and it has even been recommended as a medical treatment by doctors in Germany.

It is worth bearing in mind that several companies sell agnus castus supplements containing much higher doses than those used in scientific trials. These higher doses are not necessarily well investigated in terms of the potential for more side effects, and it is unclear whether they are more effective than the lower doses. We would generally advocate trying lower doses, as these may well be just as good.

Calcium and vitamin D

Calcium is a mineral needed by your body to regulate various chemical balances in your bloodstream, and also to keep your bones strong and prevent fractures. Vitamin D is a steroid hormone that your body needs in order to absorb the calcium from your food and store it in the body. You can get it from your diet from oily fish (such as salmon and mackerel) and eggs, and it is also generated by the skin in response to sunshine (even through sunscreen). Most people get enough as a result of everyday exposure to the sun but some women, especially those who cover up and avoid sun exposure, can be deficient in vitamin D.

It has been shown that women who are lacking in vitamin D and calcium may be more likely to develop symptoms of PMS at some stage in their life, and also that giving supplements of calcium can help ease overall symptoms. There are two possible explanations for this. Low calcium and vitamin D levels may be associated with altered patterns of changing oestrogen levels in the blood in women with PMS. Conversely, it may be because the symptoms you have with PMS are similar to symptoms from low calcium levels – for example, abdominal pains, lethargy and depression. Therefore if you already have low calcium levels you might just be pushed over the edge around the time of your period when calcium levels may naturally drop further, so that you are actually experiencing a monthly mild calcium deficiency as well as the other hormonal changes going on.

Whatever the scientific mechanisms, if you think you may be lacking in calcium, perhaps due to a low intake of dairy products and leafy vegetables such as spinach or broccoli, you may consider trying calcium supplements. It is worth remembering that calcium can't be used by your body unless you have vitamin D too. So if you don't tend to expose yourself to much sun, as well as not having much calcium in your diet, it is sensible to try a supplement that includes both vitamin D and calcium.

Three to four daily servings of low-fat dairy products are recommended in the diet. For example, you could have milk on your cereal, a yogurt at lunchtime, and a portion of cheese with sandwiches or salad. As always, all things in moderation: about a pint of milk (600 ml) is likely to provide the calcium and vitamin D you need, so don't go overboard with supplements and give yourself the problems that might result from really high calcium levels, such as constipation or kidney stones! You need about 1200 mg a day of calcium from your diet, so you should certainly not be taking more than that in supplements.

Magnesium

Magnesium is another mineral needed by the body for many different functions including preventing muscle spasms, regulating enzymes in cells and helping with healthy bones. Low levels of magnesium are very often undiagnosed, and can cause similar symptoms to PMS and low calcium – irritability, depression and muscle aches. It is found in a number of foods including chocolate, and it has been suggested that the reason we all crave chocolate is because our magnesium levels are too low.

Sounds perfect – top up your magnesium levels and never crave chocolate again! If only it were that simple. Several small studies have taken blood samples from women throughout their cycle to compare magnesium levels in women with PMS and in those with no premenstrual symptoms – and found essentially very little difference. Not so good. However, magnesium supplements have been tested as treatments for PMS, and found to significantly help with mood and also possibly with water retention. So although they may not directly ease the chocolate cravings, they may help improve the symptoms that make you feel so low that chocolate seems the only answer.

Magnesium is also believed to be quite safe, and unless you take levels outside the recommended amounts (you should not have more than 400 mg a day), you are unlikely to have many side effects. Magnesium is found in leafy vegetables, grains, nuts and seeds, although there have been reports that depletion of levels in the soil is making it more difficult to get the magnesium you need from your diet. Taking magnesium with vitamin B6 may help your body to absorb it.

Other supplements

The following have been investigated in small trials showing that they may be effective, but not enough for the RCOG to recommend their use at present: phytoestrogens, ginkgo, and pollen extract.

Phytoestrogens, also known as isoflavones, are plant hormones particularly occurring in foods such as soya, chickpeas, oats, celery and rhubarb. They may help with premenstrual migraines. Ginkgo, or the maidenhair tree, grows naturally in China. Extract from its leaves may improve blood-flow, thin the blood and protect the body from damage by free radicals (damaging particles that contribute to cell damage such as ageing and cancers). It is used for numerous disorders, particularly as a memory enhancer, though there is very limited evidence for this. A French study suggested that it could reduce breast tenderness and emotional disturbance associated with PMS.

Evening primrose oil is extracted from the seeds of evening primrose plants, which have a yellow flower which as its name suggests appears in the evenings. It is widely accepted as a good supplement for all sorts of 'woman troubles'. Although some effect has been seen with its use, in actual fact the best designed trials have not shown it to be effective. The effect of evening primrose oil, if it has any, is believed to be related to the gamma-linolenic acid (GLA) it contains. This is a type of fatty acid that has been shown by some small trials to help with breast pain, although not any other PMS symptoms. Starflower oil and blackcurrant oil also contain GLA, and therefore may be helpful for painful breasts. Starflower oil contains a higher concentration of GLA, and is consequently more expensive. There is no good-quality research to investigate its use for PMS, or how it compares to evening primrose oil.

St John's wort, *Hypericum perforatum*, is a well-known herbal preparation aimed at improving mild depression and mood symptoms. While there is a lot of anecdotal evidence for its effect on premenstrual low mood there has been very limited scientific investigation, with no large trials. There is good evidence that it helps with mild to moderate depression not related to menstruation, and may be equally as good as antidepressants, although less so for severe depression. However there is very limited evidence that it helps with PMS. In addition, there are concerns over its safety, as it is known to interact with a number of conventional medicines including antidepressants, the oral contraceptive pill, and warfarin (a blood-thinning medication sometimes prescribed for conditions such as blood clots on the legs – deep vein thrombosis). For these reasons it is not currently recommended as a treatment for PMS.

Numerous other extracts or supplements are marketed for the treatment of PMS. These include multivitamins, pollen extract (where pollen is extracted from various different flowers and mixed up to make a pollen tablet), camomile, mistletoe, valerian, kava kava, black cohosh root, and dong quai (another plant root). None of these has significant evidence to support their use, so they are not recommended by the RCOG. However, you may feel that you want to try them and make up your own mind.

Aromatherapy

Aromatherapy is the practice of using essential oils to restore emotional and physical well-being. Oils are used in different ways, from absorption by massage to hydrotherapy and inhalation. They are extracted from plants, herbs, trees and flowers, and different oils are used for specific complaints. The philosophy behind their use is linked to the idea that they affect a certain area of the brain which is involved in mood, and so as well as the potential physical healing of the plant oils themselves, they help to promote an emotional feeling of well-being, and general 'wellness'.

Specific oils are used to help with relaxation, improving concentration, overcoming insomnia, and other problems. They may be soothing, relaxing or invigorating. Most of us can remember a time when a specific smell took us straight back to a happy memory – whether it was the fresh home cooking from mum's kitchen as a child, our first-ever bunch of flowers, or the smell of a meadow when we were on a summer holiday. So it's easy to see why aromatherapy might make you feel good in the short term, but is it actually effective at overcoming real tangible symptoms from PMS?

Suggested oils for PMS are geranium, camomile and lemongrass. For depression, rose or ylang ylang could be recommended; basil for fatigue; peppermint for headaches; and lavender for insomnia, muscle pains and also headaches. There are no good-quality trials looking objectively and scientifically at the effect of aromatherapy compared with a placebo for PMS, and on this basis it is difficult to recommend it as a treatment.

However, as with most alternative therapies, it is probably something that's worth trying if it appeals to you, with the understanding that it may be totally ineffective and only have a placebo effect (you feel better because you expect to feel better, even if a treatment is actually no more effective than a Smartie). Some people are happy to use it even when they know it has only a placebo effect. Others claim that it's tremendously helpful in enabling them to relax, sleep better and feel more energized at the time of the month when they need it most.

Homoeopathy

Homoeopathy was developed in the eighteenth century and is based on the principle of 'treating like with like'. It is believed that symptoms are the body's way of fighting a disease. Therefore the symptoms of a disease can be treated by giving a tiny quantity of something that in larger quantities would cause those very symptoms; in very small quantities they stimulate the body's defence mechanisms and enable the disease to be overcome.

As a simple example, if a particular chemical was known to cause headaches, the patient might be given a very diluted version of that chemical, in order to trigger the body's defence mechanisms against headaches, and hopefully cure the root of the problem. In reality, a homoeopathic practitioner would look at the person as a whole, and treat the set of symptoms they present with, rather than just one specific treatment at a time.

The founder of homoeopathic medicine, Dr Samuel Hahneman, devised a number of principles for its practice. One of these is that the remedy required to treat a disease will cause symptoms of that disease when given to a healthy person – a principle that he developed by giving various substances to friends and family and observing which symptoms they developed. Another important principle is the idea that the more a substance is diluted, the more effective it becomes, as it loses its potential negative effects, and theoretically increases its curative effect. Thus the homoeopathic remedies you may be offered by a practitioner will contain minute amounts of the original active chemical.

Because homoeopathy is so different from conventional medicine in the way it looks at the whole person, including physical, emotional and mental aspects, it is difficult to summarize exactly what a homoeopath would give you for any particular complaint. They would usually spend some time discussing not only specific symptoms but also other aspects of your life and person. The goal is to identify how to correct those things in your life that are causing your mental, emotional or physical symptoms, thereby rectifying the specific imbalance in your life in the way that is most appropriate to you.

The scientific plausibility of homoeopathic medicine is hotly debated, especially in the medical world, but there remain many practitioners with years of experience who strongly believe that it works, and is a good alternative or adjunct to conventional medicine. There is no good scientific evidence to prove its effectiveness, although it may have some benefit over a placebo for a few conditions. There is very little evidence for its use for PMS. We leave it to you to make your mind up whether or not to investigate further and try it for yourself.

Reflexology and massage

Massage, as we all know, can be very relaxing and enjoyable. It aims to increase blood-flow, ease muscle tension, stimulate emotional well-being, and help overcome stress. It is also used by experienced practitioners to address specific symptoms and illnesses.

Reflexology is a specific type of foot massage, focusing on pressure points that are believed to be linked to other areas of the body. For example, a certain area of the foot is believed to be linked to the kidney, so stimulating this area by reflexology may help to improve blood-flow to the kidney and potentially increase its ability to clear toxins from the body, making you feel better.

Again, the scientific explanation for this therapy is not clear. There is some limited evidence from small trials that reflexology may be helpful in PMS. Although from these trials it is unknown how much of the effect was placebo and how much was actual treatment effect, you may feel that if it makes you feel relaxed and is enjoyable it doesn't really matter whether it works as a placebo or not.

Magnet therapy

Despite recent increases in advertising for magnet therapy there is no good evidence that it is effective for PMS, and scientifically there is little explanation at present for why magnets might work. Various studies have looked at the effect of magnets on blood-flow, and not found that they do very much to anything that has been measured. Magnets are marketed as potential cures for menopausal and menstrual symptoms, with many anecdotal success stories. They may well have no effect whatsoever, other than as a placebo, or they may be beneficial but just not proven yet.

If you feel you want to try this there are various options, including using a small magnet which is attached to your under-wear on the days before your period. It is claimed that it could reduce pain, bloating, water retention and other symptoms.

Other alternative therapies

These include hypnotherapy, hydrotherapy, meditation, and even crystals. We have discussed the therapies where there is some evidence that they do actually work, but there are many alternatives out there with less or no evidence for their use at all. It is easy to get taken in by wild claims and spend a lot of money on things that won't do you much good. If you want to try other therapies we would suggest you speak to your GP. Alternatively get in contact with a trusted professional or organization such as the National Association for Premenstrual Syndrome (NAPS) for more information and help to guide you through (see Useful addresses at the end of the book).

Specific concerns over safety

One of the main concerns about alternative therapies is the lack of studies to assess their safety, and particularly interactions with other medications that might be taken at the same time.

One example is St John's wort, which appears to be a good treatment for mild to moderate depression not related to PMS, but has been found to interact with a number of other treatments. For examples there have been cases of women falling pregnant while taking the oral contraceptive pill because they didn't realize that St John's wort makes the pill less effective. It also interacts with antidepressants, heart medications, and treatments for blood clots, epilepsy and HIV. Another concern about St John's wort is that there is so much variation between different products and preparations; even if you find two different brands with the same dose of St John's wort they may have different levels of other chemicals in and therefore have different effects. You should always be careful when trying new treatments, even if they are 'natural', and check with your pharmacist, doctor or alternative practitioner about any interactions with other drugs you're taking.

Another concern is light therapy, which has been suggested as a treatment for low mood, especially in the winter months. Trials investigating light therapy for PMS look at using artificial lightboxes to increase the amount of light women are exposed to. The idea of a bit of artificial extra sunshine might appeal, but there are worries that lightboxes or strong artificial light may damage the retina in the eye, potentially resulting in blindness.

It is widely accepted, however, that lack of natural light can contribute to low mood. Therefore it's probably good to make sure you get plenty of natural light. For example, walking to work, getting off the tube a stop early, taking the kids to the park or making a point to get some fresh air during your lunch break are all simple things that could help to brighten your mood. An added plus is that as long as you don't over-expose yourself and get sunburnt, the extra sunshine will make sure your vitamin D levels are topped up.

Vitamin B6 deficiency may contribute to PMS, and supplements of it have been recommended, although it is not part of current recommendations. If too high a dose is taken it can damage nerves in the hands and feet, causing tingling, numbness or pain – peripheral neuropathy. A maximum dose of 10 mg a day should be taken, so if you decide to take supplements make sure you don't exceed this.

Tables 7.1 and 7.2 below and opposite provide a summary of treatments for specific symptoms, and the evidence currently available for them.

Table 7.1 Psychological and emotional symptoms

Symptom	Treatment	Evidence
Low mood/ depression	Exercise	No clear evidence from trials, but generally recommended – likely to be beneficial
	Antidepressants	Good
	Saffron	One small but good placebo-controlled trial
	Vitamin B6 (pyridoxine)	Limited evidence, poor-quality trials
Irritability and anger	Agnus castus	Good
	Pollen extract	Limited, may help after 2–4 months' treatment
Poor memory/ concentration	Ginkgo	Very limited although widely marketed for this
Insomnia	Reducing caffeine	Good

Table 7.2 Physical symptoms

Symptom	Treatment	Evidence
Abdominal cramps	Magnesium	Good
Bloating and water retention	Dietary changes – reduced salt intake, increased water and fibre	Limited but generally recommended by health professionals
	Vitamin B6	Poor-quality trials, may help
Breast tenderness	Agnus castus	Good
	Reducing caffeine	Limited, but may help
	Evening primrose oil and possibly starflower oil	Limited evidence. May be effective for cyclical breast pain
	Ginkgo	Limited but may help

(continued)

Table 7.2 Physical symptoms (*continued*)

Symptom	Treatment	Evidence
Headache	Agnus castus	Good
	Isoflavones (phytoestrogens)	Limited evidence, may help relieve premenstrual migraines
General symptoms	Calcium and Vitamin D	Good evidence for improving overall PMS; not proven for any specific symptom
	Reflexology	Small, poorly controlled trial – very limited evidence; marketed for most PMS symptoms

Summary

- Treatment for PMS depends on an individual's symptoms, preferences and circumstances.
- Treatment can be *conservative* (lifestyle changes you can make); *medical* (treatments a doctor can give you); *alternative* (non-medical treatments or therapies).
- Lifestyle changes address diet, exercise, weight loss, stress, smoking.
- Medical treatments include a newer version of the pill, painkillers.
- The best evidence for alternative therapies is for agnus castus, calcium and vitamin D, magnesium.
- Numerous other alternative therapies are available.

8

Severe PMS/PMDD

The Royal College of Obstetricians and Gynaecologists (RCOG) recognizes that some women suffer from a severe form of PMS. If you're unfortunate enough to have a GP who doesn't seem to believe you, or makes you feel that it's all in your head and nothing to do with your hormones, you can tell them otherwise – before you change GP. The RCOG suggests the same initial approach as for less severe PMS. The severity of symptoms should be properly assessed with a symptom diary, so that the key problems to be addressed can be recognized.

The spectrum of severity of PMS is defined as follows: mild PMS 'does not interfere with personal/social and professional life'; moderate PMS 'interferes with personal/social and professional life but [you are] still able to function and interact, although maybe sub-optimally'; and severe PMS makes you 'unable to interact personally/socially/professionally', withdrawing from 'social and professional activities'; or it is 'treatment resistant'.

Premenstrual dysphoric disorder (PMDD) is essentially the same as severe PMS, but with more specific criteria for symptoms. Some people use the term to refer more generally to severe emotional or psychological symptoms. It is a term not recognized by the RCOG; they refer to it as a research term, adopted in the US for referring to severe PMS.

Every woman should be given advice about lifestyle changes such as diet, exercise and reducing stress levels before any treatment is started, as even the worst symptoms can sometimes be managed with simple measures. Some women suffer with psychological symptoms, which may be severe enough to require referral to a psychiatrist. It is important to realize that psychiatric illnesses are reported to exist just in the premenstrual phase, and that if you suffer terribly with your PMS – even having severe depression, feeling suicidal or having symptoms of schizophrenia only at that time of the month – you are not alone, and a psychiatrist may actually be able to help significantly. If a symptom diary is kept then these symptoms can be assessed early and you can be referred to the best person to help you.

While most women should, in an ideal world, be able to have their treatment coordinated by their GP, in women with severe PMS it is suggested that a multidisciplinary team (MDT) is very helpful. This team comprises both medical and non-medical staff, often including doctors (a GP and/or hospital gynaecologist), psychiatrist or psychologist, dietician, counsellor, and district nurse. The team will be able to address the different aspects that may be contributing to your symptoms, as well as the different treatments you may want to try. An 'integrated' approach is advised, which means that not only do you see your doctor or members of your MDT, but you also try out the lifestyle changes suggested and try alternative therapies alongside the medical therapies if you want to. Medical and alternative therapies shouldn't be viewed as one or the other, but as complementing each other, according to what each woman wants to try.

Medical therapies

The idea of medical therapy in severe PMS is either to overcome severe psychological, emotional or psychiatric symptoms with appropriately used antidepressants or behavioural therapy, or to stop ovulation (either medically or surgically), so that the body's oestrogen and progesterone balance can be controlled.

After confirming the diagnosis of severe PMS, a suggested first-line approach of treatment is to try combining exercise with counselling or cognitive behavioural therapy. A new generation of oral contraceptive pill or monthly antidepressants just in the premenstrual phase are alternatives. Alternatively all three could be tried one by one or together. If these are unsuccessful the second step might be to try hormone therapy with oestrogen patches. The antidepressant dose could be increased or used continuously through your cycle.

However, if none of these measures helps, a stronger hormonal treatment could be tried – a GnRH analogue, or 'gonadorelin'. This is a man-made version of the gonadotrophin-releasing hormone (GnRH) from the hypothalamus discussed in Chapter 3 which causes the pituitary gland to release luteinizing hormone (LH) and follicle-stimulating hormone (FSH). Rather than causing the release of the gonadotrophin hormones, as occurs in the natural cycle, the GnRH analogue overwhelms the pituitary gland and totally blocks the production of these sex hormones, thus preventing the menstrual cycle from taking place. You therefore need to take hormone replacement therapy (HRT) to regulate exactly what's going on with all those muddled hormone levels. This is a kind of medical way of taking your ovaries out of the picture.

The absolute last-line treatment, if none of the above works, would be to have a hysterectomy, also removing the ovaries, and afterwards taking HRT until the time of the menopause.

At each step along the way of medical treatment, any alternative therapies can, of course, be tried. It would be wise to try just one therapy at a time so that you can see which treatment is successful.

Antidepressants

There is good evidence from a large review of a number of research trials that antidepressants are effective for treating both the psychological and physical symptoms of PMS – in particular, selective serotonin reuptake inhibitors (SSRIs), which include drugs such as fluoxetine (Prozac) and citalopram. Your GP should prescribe these only if he or she has a special interest in women's health and is familiar with prescribing antidepressants for PMS. If not, your GP should refer you to a gynaecologist or psychiatrist, whichever is most appropriate.

It is believed that since low levels of serotonin may contribute to PMS, those antidepressants that stop the brain from storing it away again after it is released (that is, prevent its reuptake), allow the serotonin to stay in the brain a bit longer, hence boosting your mood and easing symptoms. They can be effective for anxiety and depression, as well as some physical symptoms (although not headaches). This may be because when your mood is low you are less able to tolerate physical discomfort, so if your general mood and well-being are improved, it can help you to deal with symptoms that wouldn't bother you on a normal day, but become too much when you're tired and feeling down.

You may be concerned about the side effects and consequences of taking antidepressants. The commonest side effects are nausea, which can be severe but usually improves within a week of treatment, insomnia, and reduced sex drive; withdrawal symptoms may be experienced if the medication is taken for several months and then stopped abruptly. To reduce these symptoms and also to avoid the problems of dependence leading to withdrawal, antidepressants can be taken just in the last one to two weeks of your cycle, before your period. There is evidence that this is just as effective as taking them constantly, it reduces side effects, and you can stop them without having to taper the dose. The benefits from these antidepressants are sufficiently well recognized for the RCOG to recommend that they be considered as one of the first-line options in medical management of severe PMS.

Counselling

Various types of counselling exist. You may find it helpful simply to talk through what you're experiencing with someone outside your situation, who can listen impartially and allow you the time and space to get things into perspective. This can be done alongside whatever treatment you might be using, and may be available either through your GP, or a private organization.

Cognitive behavioural therapy (CBT) is a specific type of indepth counselling, which is actually considered a treatment in itself. It is a combination of cognitive therapy and behavioural therapy. Cognitive therapy is based on the idea that the way you perceive yourself can have just as much or more effect on how you feel about an event or circumstance as the event itself. It aims to identify thinking errors, and people's assumptions about themselves and their world (their 'cognitive schema'). These errors and schema can then be addressed and corrected to enable you to better approach your circumstances and subsequent events, with a healthy outlook.

Behavioural therapy is the practical side of the coin, focusing on recognizing unwanted behaviours. It involves various treatments including relaxation training (breathing and muscle exercises), response prevention (helping you learn to control and stop responses that you don't want, such as screaming at the kids when they leave dirty plates around *again!*), exposure therapy (gradually becoming familiar with situations/things that cause you psychological distress), and active scheduling (planning specific tasks to help overcome particular difficulties). This may sound very technical, but can be tremendously helpful.

A trial comparing antidepressants (fluoxetine), CBT and a combination of the two found that they were equally effective for severe PMS. Six months of antidepressants improved symptoms more quickly, but ten sessions of CBT had a more lasting effect a year after treatment. They were equally effective, but combining them didn't have any further benefit. On this basis, the RCOG recommend that CBT should be routinely considered in severe PMS. It is conducted by a clinical psychologist, and should be available to every woman where appropriate.

If you feel that this would be helpful to you it's worth speaking to your GP, who should be able to help. Unfortunately the usual funding issues in the NHS may mean that it is not available at your local practice, or you may be put on a long waiting list. Although things are improving, you might need to be persistent. A typical course of cognitive behavioural therapy would involve ten weekly sessions, and may be a good idea if you feel your PMS involves lots of emotional turmoil, and you don't want to take antidepressants.

Oestrogen

The use of the oral contraceptive pill is discussed in Chapter 7. An alternative in severe PMS is oestrogen given either as an implant (under the skin, usually on your arm) or by weekly patches. There is good evidence that this slow release of oestrogen is effective in reducing symptoms. The only problem with it is that you can't have oestrogen on its own for too long, as it increases the risk of endometrial cancer (affecting the lining of the womb). Some progesterone needs to be given as well, unless you have had a hysterectomy, to balance out the oestrogen and prevent this.

Progesterone can be either taken in tablet form during part of your cycle, or given directly into the womb by the Mirena coil. This is like the traditional contraceptive coil, except that as well as providing contraception by preventing implantation of an embryo, it releases small amounts of progesterone locally into the womb. This may initially cause some PMS-type symptoms and irregular bleeding, but these usually settle down so that the oestrogen patch can work on your symptoms, while the coil protects the lining of the womb (also providing contraception, if this is necessary). Some doctors would suggest using progesterone pessaries in the vagina instead of using the Mirena, and this is something you could discuss with your doctor if you felt that would be better for you.

The risk of endometrial cancer from this type of oestrogen treatment is thought to be small when used with progesterone, but there isn't any clear data on the exact risk, and there is potentially an increased risk of breast cancer, although this is also unclear. If you have a family history of breast cancer you should discuss these risks with your doctor before starting treatment.

The other point to bear in mind is that the patches or implant used to treat PMS do not provide contraception as well, so if you are not using the coil and need contraception you must make sure you use alternative protection.

Steroids

Danazol is a steroid with anti-oestrogen and anti-progesterone properties. It is licensed for use in endometriosis, but has also been shown to be highly effective in treating PMS, although it has not been officially licensed for this use in the UK. Some women report significant improvements with it, particularly for breast tenderness.

However, as you might expect, taking steroids is not without its risks. There are several side effects associated with its use, including nausea, dizziness, skin reactions, and fatigue, among others. The main concern with its use is the potential for virilization, a process whereby a woman develops certain male characteristics, such as facial hair, acne, or a deep voice or even enlargement of the clitoris. This can be very distressing and may occasionally be irreversible.

Danazol could be something to try if you have exhausted all the hormonal treatments and nothing seems to help and your symptoms are becoming unbearable; it is clearly not a first resort. Despite sometimes being very effective, because of the possibility of serious side effects it would not be recommended by doctors other than in very severe cases, and after trying other therapies. It may be taken only in the second half of your cycle, which reduces the risk of side effects, and should not be used for more than six months.

GnRH analogues

Again, these are not a first resort. But if other treatments have been unsuccessful you may wish to try gonadotrophin-releasing hormone (GnRH) analogues. GnRH is a hormone released in the hypothalamus (in the brain) to stimulate the production of oestrogen and progesterone via the pituitary gland and ovaries, as discussed in Chapter 3. GnRH analogues are man-made copies of this hormone, which effectively tire out the production mechanisms, stopping your body from producing oestrogen and progesterone and so stopping your cycle altogether. If you definitely have cyclical symptoms, and therefore an accurate diagnosis of PMS, this medication should significantly reduce your symptoms, especially the physical ones.

Sounds ideal! The only problem is that your body does actually need oestrogen for other purposes that have nothing to do with fertility or menstruation. You may get symptoms of the menopause with this medication (the classic hot flushes, for example) as it in effect causes a medically induced menopause. Without oestrogen, you struggle to keep the calcium you need in your bones and therefore also risk developing osteoporosis – thinning of the bones – which puts you at high risk of fractures. For these reasons, GnRH analogues should not be taken in the long term; their use should be limited to six months and combined with hormone replacement therapy (HRT) to put back a balanced amount of the hormones your body needs.

If your symptoms are unbearable, and this is the only treatment that helps, your doctor may consider continuing with it for longer, in which case you would need to be particularly careful regarding your diet, exercise, avoiding smoking and having regular (yearly) bone scans to monitor your risk of osteoporosis. Alternatively, if totally stopping your periods really makes a difference to your life, and you're certain that you don't want any or any more children, you could consider a hysterectomy with removal of the ovaries.

Hysterectomy

It may seem extreme, and is not often required, but surgery may be an option if your PMS is significantly affecting your life and no treatment is helping. Ideally, it shouldn't be considered unless you have tried GnRH analogues, as they produce the same kind of effect as removing your womb and ovaries; so if your symptoms have not resolved by taking them, they may not resolve with surgery. Removing your womb and ovaries will permanently stop the production of oestrogen and progesterone, stop your cycle, and therefore by definition stop your premenstrual symptoms. The majority of women who undergo this surgery are very happy with the outcome, so if you feel it may be for you, you should definitely discuss it with your doctor.

There are risks as well as benefits with every surgery, and a hysterectomy can be a big operation, so it is important that you consider these before going ahead. Your doctor would explain all the medical risks of the procedure, such as bleeding, serious blood clots and infection, but something that often isn't discussed is the emotional effect it can have. Some women describe a sense of emotional loss after a hysterectomy, which may be quite unexpected. They sometimes feel that they have lost a part of what makes them a woman, and this can take time to come to terms with.

The operation is, of course, totally irreversible, so the worst thing you can possibly do is have a hysterectomy because you're so distressed by your PMS, and then when it goes away decide that you and your partner want to try for another baby! It is also worth bearing in mind that if you have a hysterectomy while you're still relatively young you need to take hormone replacement therapy to avoid the risks associated with low oestrogen levels, such as fragile bones from osteoporosis. For some women this is an ideal solution, while others can't bear the thought of taking more medications.

If, having considered the potential negative aspects of surgery, you still feel it is the best option for you, then as long as your symptoms are definitely premenstrual (and therefore unlikely to be due to anything other than PMS) if all goes well you should be very satisfied with your treatment.

Summary

Some of the medical therapies described sound quite extreme, with potentially horrible side effects. The descriptions are not meant to put you off or make you feel negative about the medical options for PMS but to help you make informed decisions. Some treatments might have only limited effects but hardly any problems associated with them, while others may be extremely effective but risk worse side effects. While you may try a therapy with certain potential side effects, you will not necessarily be affected; you could have your PMS cured by the first medicine you take, or you may find you need to try several treatments. Some readers will not have been to see a GP at all, while others will feel they've tried so many therapies they don't know what to do next. It is for you to decide what you do and don't want to try, with the information you need and the help of your doctor.

Support networks

It is absolutely crucial that anyone experiencing any medical or psychological distress has the support they need, whether it's from friends, family or specific organizations. This applies just as much to PMS as any other situation. It may be that you feel your family or those around you struggle to understand, or that you feel guilty for what you put them through every month. It is incredibly common to feel alone, as if no one else could possibly be as ill, or as crazy as you are every month. However, there are thousands of women suffering from exactly the same condition, who may be feeling just as alone.

There are many ways to help deal with this sense of being alone. It can be really valuable to spend time speaking to your partner and/or family, discussing your monthly symptoms with them and working out ways to help the family cope better at those times.

They may need the opportunity to tell you the things about your symptoms that they struggle with, and you can discuss what they can do to help.

For example, if they're old enough, you could ask your children to make their own packed lunch in the evening for one week a month, to avoid the early morning stresses when you're tired, irritable and don't want to argue with them about what to put in their sandwiches. You could explain to friends that during your premenstrual week you'll need some time to yourself, so you would prefer to put off meeting up for coffee or social occasions until the week after. It may help to plan positive events that you feel will lift your mood and not demand too much energy in that week.

Either way, it is important to be honest with those around you. Although it might be difficult to hear how your symptoms affect them if they're equally honest with you, it may help to address and reduce frictions caused by your PMS, which have previously been building up, or seemed insurmountable. Cliché though it is, communication really is crucial.

Sometimes talking to friends and family just isn't enough, especially if they don't seem to understand what's wrong with you, or why you can't just 'fix up' and pull yourself together. Support groups exist around the country and can be totally invaluable. It's often tremendously helpful to talk with women who are not that unlike you, have the same stresses to cope with, and are dealing with similar symptoms. They may suggest different ways of coping, or it may just reassure you to realize how common PMS is, and that it doesn't have to rule your life.

The National Association for Premenstrual Syndrome is a great resource for information and support, and may help you with finding contacts and local support groups. You may find it takes a lot of effort to pluck up the courage to go to a meeting with people you don't know and talk about your problems, but many women find these groups positive and incredibly worthwhile. You might even want to start up a support group yourself if there isn't one in your area, and help others who are affected too.

Another important aspect of PMS is the effect it has on your work. Some women simply cannot function well enough to go to work for a day or even a week before their period. This is extremely difficult to deal with if your employer is not very understanding. You can feel that you're letting the team down or that everyone perceives you as lazy, calling in sick more often than you should. Clearly this can't go on indefinitely, not turning up to work for one week in four, so it is important to speak to your boss, or occupational health department if you have one, to discuss the situation. They should work with you to formulate reasonable goals and a plan of action. This may involve a lighter workload during that week, or planning to have certain days off so that your boss knows what they can and can't expect of you. If you're upfront, hopefully they will be reasonable with you too – much better than going in feeling that the office is resenting you, or that you aren't achieving what you want to at work.

The most important thing is not to give up: find what's right for you, and if you feel that it's getting too much to handle, *get help*. We hope this book will be a useful resource in helping you to do that.

Summary

- A multidisciplinary team of different professionals may include doctors, a psychiatrist, dietician, counsellor and district nurse.
- Effective treatments include antidepressants, cognitive behavioural therapy (CBT), oestrogen therapy, GnRH analogues, Danazol (a steroid), hysterectomy.
- Medical treatments may have side effects to consider:
  - Oestrogen does not provide contraception; some form of progesterone is needed.
  - Long-term GnRH analogues can cause bone-thinning.
  - Danazol therapy can have irreversible serious side effects.
  - Removal of the womb and ovaries can have a significant fertility and emotional impact and is a last resort, but can be very successful if done appropriately.
- Support from friends, family, support groups and professionals is crucial.

9

The male perspective

This chapter is dedicated to those men who are affected, directly or indirectly, as a result of PMS. It has been suggested that some men living with women with PMS may have cyclical mood symptoms themselves, but since there is clearly no menstruation going on in a man's body, this is certainly not the same thing as PMS. It may be possible that men themselves are afflicted with some kind of cyclical change in hormone levels that affects their mood, or that the pheromones or hormones given out by menstruating women may unwittingly affect a man's emotional state.

Nevertheless, it remains difficult to discount the probability that men are grumpy or miserable at 'that time of the month' because they're simply fed up of dealing with, or trying to be patient with, the woman they live with when it's 'that time of the month' for her. While men may not experience any cyclical change, they will certainly be affected by their partner's moods, and we as women really do need to understand this, and perhaps try to gain a better understanding of their views on things, and how best to help them understand us.

Effect on relationships

In January 2009 the BBC reported a case of relationship breakdown because of the severity of a woman's PMS. She was subject to intolerable mood swings for at least ten days every month. Her husband eventually became so frustrated and distressed that he walked out. She has now had treatment for her PMS, and they have fortunately been able to work through their problems with relationship counselling, but their story is not unique. There is no accurate data on the number of couples affected by PMS, but the number is likely to be huge. It is surely impossible to live with someone with severe symptoms every month without it putting at least some degree of strain on your relationship.

Women often feel misunderstood, frustrated, poorly supported or even guilty about the effects their symptoms have on their loved ones. Partners may struggle to understand or relate to all this, feeling frustrated or angry that their woman can't pull herself together, or guilty for not being able to help. Month after month this combination has the potential to lead to a couple avoiding each other, not talking about important issues, arguing, or simply drifting apart. In particular, PMS can seriously affect a couple's sex life for many reasons, including its effect on sex drive, their emotional connection, and physical discomfort making sex less pleasurable during the premenstrual time. Recognizing and addressing all these relationship issues means that they can potentially be avoided or resolved. Some women actually report increased sex drive premenstrually, and working through the problems caused by PMS can result in a much healthier and more enjoyable relationship than you may have had in the past.

Being on the receiving end

For partners of women with PMS, feelings of frustration, confusion, anger, empathy and guilt are all possible. When their partners are suffering from irritability or low mood men may feel they can't get anything right; they get fed up, or even give up trying. One woman reported that her PMS causes so much angst in her household that she and her husband refer to it as 'sin'. It is clear that PMS must be having a significant effect on that household!

Men can feel resentful that they have to take on so many other chores when their partners are less capable than usual. It's easy for him to wonder why his woman can't understand that *he* has work stresses, is tired and doesn't want to come home late to deal with the things she usually does, while she sits and mopes in front of the TV.

Differences between men and women

In her song 'The Best Damn Thing', popular Australian singer Avril Lavigne complains that he can't understand why at that time of the month she doesn't want to hold his hand. In many areas, and particularly PMS, this seems to be a very common theme in many a relationship: 'he doesn't understand'. If men did more to try and understand what's happening when PMS affects their women, and perhaps if women did more to help them understand rather than just moan at them for not doing so, maybe some of the upset and frustrations that can be caused in a relationship could be eased.

It's now widely accepted that, as described in the famous book by John Gray, figuratively speaking 'men are from Mars, women are from Venus'. There will always be intrinsic, unchangeable differences between the sexes. However, as history has shown us, even some of the most glaring differences in culture and viewpoint can eventually be bridged and overcome. It may be that a compromise on both sides to understand the effects of PMS on a woman herself, as well as on those around her, can help to bring about more of the mutual understanding that enables couples to work through the most disabling and distressing premenstrual symptoms.

The natural differences in men's and women's approaches to problem-solving may contribute to and exacerbate relationship problems around PMS time. As a rule men want to solve everything sensibly, but often when we're premenstrual we can't even define the problem to be solved, let alone think logically about the best thing to do about it. Other women will usually understand (to some degree) when we need to be listened to, allowed to rant or left in peace. Unfortunately, well-meaning men will often try to step in and suggest solutions; these will naturally be met with a less than positive response if all a woman wants to do is moan or have her problems acknowledged.

One of the big problems with PMS is that many women find it seriously affects their reasoning and rational thinking, making it harder for them to define specific problems, and making multiple small problems seem much more significant and indistinguishable. For example, 'the ironing pile looks horrible and needs to be done, we've only got one more day's milk in the fridge and my boss is piling on the pressure to sort this file out' can turn from separate, surmountable tasks to a sea of stress that seems to keep washing over you so fast you can't think straight. Therefore you may feel generally more stressed or irritable without being able to pinpoint why; so when a guy comes along and helpfully suggests you get on with the ironing while he goes to get some milk, it can feel as if he's trivializing all your stress. As you become more aware of yourself and your reactions, as well as those of the man in your life, you can consciously start to recognize those times when you're being frustrated with each other as a result of your PMS, rather than any problem with your relationship itself.

Interestingly, there is a suggestion that women in same-sex relationships suffer less PMS, and feel more supported by their partners if they do – a statistic that will probably make the men feel even worse!

PMS at work – does it still contribute to the glass ceiling?

In the workplace, dealing with your PMS can be extremely difficult. Discussing it can be even more difficult, as there seems to be such a fine line between male chauvinism, with its total lack of understanding of the female perspective, and aggressive feminism with its inability to see things from the perspective of a man. The ideal, as with any other issues that affect men and women differently, is to try and take into account a balanced perspective of both points of view.

The last thing any woman wants to do is admit incompetence at her job because of hormones – 'how will they ever respect me again?' Conversely, it can be desperately frustrating for a man if he feels that the women in the office are pulling their weight for only three weeks out of four while he has to put in all his effort all the time. Men may feel that it's not fair that women get away with doing less and blaming it on their hormones. Of course, this all-too-common stereotype is usually not the case; there are lazy women just as much as there are lazy men, but most people who want to keep their job and do well in their career will work as much as they possibly can, and some women genuinely do struggle to perform at work at that time of the month.

There's no easy answer, and obviously the goal is to find the right remedy for your PMS so that you can get on with your job without having to dose up with strong painkillers, or come in to work feeling half-dead for one week every month. In the meantime there's no reason why men as well as other women can't be supportive and helpful. It will always be hard for people who don't have PMS to understand, but showing that you really do work your best when you're able to and that you only need time off when you genuinely are suffering, is the best you can do as a woman. The bottom line is, if your PMS is genuinely so bad that you can't go to work you should look at it in the same way as any other illness until it improves and you're able to cope again.

If you're seriously struggling to work through every month because of your PMS and you find there's little support at work, you may need to talk frankly with your occupational health department. For some women their PMS is so bad that they have only one or two weeks of normality a month, and have had to give up work altogether. Fortunately this is the exception, and the majority of women are able to find a workable solution. But if things do get this bad, it is just as hard as with any non-hormone-related illness that stops you earning the money you need to pay your mortgage; so from the man's perspective, understanding the severity and significance of PMS on some women should help to make it no more (or less) irritating than when colleagues require sick leave for other reasons – from flu to broken bones or depression.

Trying to understand some of the impact on your male as well as female colleagues of taking time off due to PMS may help you to maintain relationships with them when you go back to work. But it is important not to struggle on, feeling guilty that others might suffer because of your illness – you need to cope with it for you more than for anyone else.

Men don't have cyclical illnesses, but they do get ill, and whether they're the type to soldier on or not, they sometimes have to appreciate that the body simply isn't always as strong as the mind wants it to be. You may need to be flexible in planning your workload to alleviate the premenstrual stress, but since it can be predictable, it may actually be easier to work around than some unpredictable complaints that make it hard for men to work to their full capacity.

The 'silver lining'

On the other hand, some men may unwittingly be glad PMS exists – it gives them an excuse for not understanding women, and also for not having to ask why a woman isn't her normal self. Believing that most female miseries can be attributed to hormones may well absolve a guy from having to ask or try to understand what's wrong, as he can happily accept that he'll never get to the bottom of it or be able to relate to it – so it's best not to try! It might also be a good excuse for offering to go out (down the pub with some mates) and leave her some space. In some cases this might be just what a couple need to avoid conflict at that time, as long as he doesn't decide to leg it every time she's looking a bit down.

Pre-MANstrual syndrome

Simonides (556–468 BC), the Greek lyric poet, wrote a poem on the pedigree of women. Here are a few excerpts from his writings:

> ...God made from the wicked vixen, a woman who knows all things. Whether bad or good, nothing escapes her notice; for often she calls a good thing bad and a bad thing good; her mood keeps changing ...

> ... one day she smiles and beams with joy; the next day, though, she is unbearable to lay eyes on or to come near to; at that time she rages unapproachably ... proving implacable and repulsive to everyone ...

Women reading this may find it both profoundly distressing and utterly shocking; if you're a man then you possibly couldn't agree more! So, even in ancient times, it seems that men were just as perplexed at women's premenstrual behaviour and it seems that Simonides has provided men with the much sought-after licence that allows men to coin themselves as the innocent victims of PMS.

So, 'pre-manstrual syndrome' – generally defined as 'the protective reflex of a male when his mate is suffering from premenstrual syndrome'! Is it simply a case of male 'me-too-ism' or are men affected by hormonal fluctuations too? Well, since the normal biorhythm of men does not follow the same cyclical pattern as their female counterparts, it is not surprising that at present there is no research to support the case for 'pre-manstrual syndrome'.

Tips for guys

Although women suffer *with* PMS, we also understand that men suffer *because* of it. Below is a short list of helpful hints to try to ease the difficulties of 'that time of the month' for you and your partner. But to start with, <PMSbuddy.com> is an online 'PMS reminder' aimed at males. It aims to 'Save relationships, one month at a time!' The website was created in 2007, and works by sending email notifications in the lead-up to PMS!

It's not always easy being a man around hormonal women, so here are seven survival tips.

1 *Acknowledge that it may happen*, and be prepared for it. Get out of the house if you need to – plan some nights out with the lads if you think it's best to be out of the way. But if you think a few wild nights out are likely to upset her or make her more insecure, try scheduling them for a more appropriate time.

2 *Expect that she may be a bit unreasonable* just before her period's due. Arguing at this time can often turn into an argument for argument's sake rather than actually resolving anything, so try to avoid conflict and be patient (but don't patronize her). You don't have to be a doormat (not many women like them) but a bit of extra compromise at that time of the month could go a long way. If you've got a decent woman she should appreciate it, even if not straight away.

3 *Don't expect to always know what she's upset about*. Most of the time hormonal women don't know why they're upset themselves, and after snapping at you for not taking the rubbish out, or feeding the cat, or whatever else it is, she may well burst into tears and just need a cuddle. Don't argue, don't always try to make sense of it, just be there. When she's feeling better you can broach the subject of why she was cross with you for not doing the only household chore she's never let you do before, or not booking the cinema tickets she said she didn't want ... If she's upset about something that really is significant to her, it will probably be easier to talk it through at a less emotional time.

4 *Try to be understanding.* If she tells you to leave her alone some-times she means it and wants some space; sometimes she wants you to let her moan and just not interrupt. Sometimes she doesn't know herself. But you can try. If your female partner suffers more from physical symptoms seek out what remedies best ease them, be sympathetic, and look after her until she's feeling better. She'll do it for you when you're ill! Remember that PMS is not who she is – it's something that affects you both; it may be really helpful for her just to realize that you love her for her, even when she feels horrible.

5 *Don't be a girl.* Girls notoriously complain that it's not what you say but how you say it. While we all know this can be the case, don't be offended if she snaps at you because she wants fish fingers and not waffles. That may actually be all there is to it.

6 *Be honest.* If you feel fed up with her doing something specific, say so, as sensitively as possible. It's better to resolve something if it can be resolved than let it fester, but do try and pick your moment carefully. If you're honest with her she should be honest with you.

7 *See it as a positive opportunity* to do the manly, caring thing, and look after your female partner. Bring home some of her favourite biscuits or make her a special hot chocolate when you can see she's feeling a bit frayed. Even if she's grumpy and unappre-ciative at the time she'll remember how sweet you've been when she snaps out of it and feels normal again the following week – and love you more for it.

If you're in a long-term relationship try to look at PMS as some-thing you work through together. Until you find the solution to ease or relieve your symptoms, you and your partner can work out ways to help each other cope, just as you do with other issues. Even if things seem really bad right now, being in a relationship is about partnership, sharing problems, and sorting them out together – just like you will with work or financial problems, children, health issues, and the false teeth and Zimmer frames when you both get older. At some point you might look back together and laugh and cry about the dramas and pain you went through when PMS was a big problem in your lives. It may seem idealistic, and it's not always easy, but it's easier to weather the storm if you face it together.

Lastly, a few stories from the men

I work in a salon with all girls and they're not shy about times of the month. Sometimes I don't know if I don't want to go to work or just laugh about it. They get so grumpy, knock stuff over, get stressed about the tiniest thing. It's funny really.

Mike's been married for over 20 years and has given up worrying about it:

I let her go to bed if she wants and just get on with things. It's less hassle!

Some slightly less understanding men:

I don't see why women can just not bother and expect us to do their job for them just because of some stupid hormones. Sort it out or get another job.

It's imaginary, isn't it?!

That's exactly why a woman shouldn't be president: wrong time of the month and she might press the nuclear button.

Sometimes I've genuinely wanted to kill my wife. I shouldn't say it but if she hadn't gone to the doctor and started sorting it out one of us would have left.

'UB' was slightly more animated in his response:

Women are as nutty regardless of whether they're PMSing or not!

Similarly 'MA', who has three sisters, said:

We are the victims here! ... Women are inherently irrational any time of the year, month, day, hour or second! It's inexcusable.

Peh! PMS?! PM – what?! PMS and the three little bears? PMS drove Little Red Riding Hood crazy and she evolved into a wolf! ... PMS is a fairy-tale friend!

But they're not all like that. Craig has stuck by his fianceé when she's been too uncomfortable to go out or do much, and he thinks it's made them stronger.

We deal with it now; she lets me know when she's due and we just get on with it. She looks out for me when I'm ill, and I try and take care of her. I think it's a bit better than it used to be. She took some tablets for a while but I don't think she takes anything now. If she's feeling rough we just stay in and cuddle up in front of the TV.

I don't get what all the fuss is about. None of the girls I work with has ever had a problem. Sometimes there's a bit of banter if some-one's more moody than usual but I don't know if it's really PMS.

Imran has been married for two years:

PMS represents premenstrual stress for the men of this world in a relationship. The strange hormonal ways of women are still a mystery to men worldwide despite the length of time they have spent with their other half. The monthly cycle represents a time where logic is thrown out the window, where men must accept guilt for the things they have done and even for the things they may not have done in order to avoid earache or in some cases physical violence. In my own personal experience I have found that nodding your head, saying 'yes' to everything she asks and avoiding any form of response to the 'hairdryer' treatment extends the periods of marital bliss that are otherwise in place during the other three weeks.

'ST', who has been married for three years, counts himself as one of the lucky few:

I'm actually really lucky and my Mrs doesn't get any symptoms nor does she take it out on me! It just goes to show that not all women get it and so shouldn't use it as an excuse to cause us misery!

Jeremy talks about his experiences when he was a final-year medical student in Bristol:

In my final year at university I moved into a house with eight girls, myself the only boy. I think they wanted me for tasks like killing spiders and reaching for things on top of particularly tall cupboards. To me living in a house full of attractive women was pretty much the achievement of what I had envisioned when applying to university. The trouble with trying to describe any experiences I might have had with premenstrual syndrome is that I obviously had little knowledge or interest in this area of my housemates' lives. Furthermore, trying to ascribe patterns of behaviour to this cause has traditionally been seen as a bit chauvinist. One thing that you learn early on in life is that there is nothing that annoys a girl more than telling her that she is a victim of her hormones, so this opinion given here is nothing more than unashamedly prejudiced supposition.

It was certainly the case that none of the girls would admit that they suffered from PMS. Even if there are biologically valid reasons why they might feel more tired or stressed because of periods there was a strong resistance to any idea that this may have been an underlying cause. My friends had counselled me before entering the house that I should expect havoc at certain times of the month when all their periods synchronize. I didn't find this to be at all true, however.

Some of the girls had no predictably regular behaviour down-turns, whereas others did have them but at different times of the month. At these times boyfriend arguments increased, emotions became more labile, and fake tan grew thicker to compensate for a decrease in self-esteem. As I am a big fan of having an easy life I found the way to cope with this was to agree with whoever was displaying these types of symptoms. The other type of reaction I observed was that some girls seemed to withdraw from house activities for a few days, remaining very quiet at these times. I'm sure that a number of relationship break-ups coincided with this time of the month. In summary I cannot for sure attribute these activities to PMS but I have a suspicion it may have been a con-tributing factor.

Summary

- PMS can indirectly affect men as it affects the women around them.
- The effect on relationships can be significant.
- Communication and an effort to understand each other are crucial.
- Don't underestimate the effect PMS may have on your man – or he may start complaining of pre-MANstrual syndrome – the word is out . . .

Useful addresses

British Dietetic Association
5th Floor, Charles House
148/9 Great Charles Street
Queensway
Birmingham B3 3HT
Tel.: 0121 200 8080
Fax: 0121 200 8081
Email: info@bda.uk.com
Website: www.bda.uk.com

The association offers good practical advice for healthy eating, and also provides a factsheet on eating to help to relieve PMS.

Food Standards Agency
UK Headquarters
Aviation House
125 Kingsway
London WC2B 6NH
Helpline: 020 7276 8829
Email: helpline@foodstandards.gsi.gov.uk
Website: www.food.gov.uk

Northern Ireland office
10c Clarendon Road
Belfast BT1 3BG
Tel.: 02890 417700
Email: infofsani@foodstandards.gsi.gov.uk

Food Standards Agency Scotland
6th Floor, St Magnus House
25 Guild Street
Aberdeen AB11 6NJ
Tel.: 01224 285100
Email: scotland@foodstandards.gsi.gov.uk

Wales office
11th Floor, South Gate House
Wood Street
Cardiff CF10 1EW
Tel.: 02920 678999
Email: wales@foodstandards.gsi.gov.uk

The FSA is the government's independent department for public health

related to food. It has information on government recommendations for
healthy eating.

National Association for Premenstrual Syndrome (NAPS)
41 Old Road
East Peckham
Kent TN12 5AP
Tel.: 0870 777 2178
Fax: 0870 777 2178
Website: www.pms.org.uk

This charity offers high-quality, professional advice to sufferers and also
healthcare professionals working with people with PMS. It has a useful
online diary for charting symptoms.

Premenstrual Society (PREMSOC)
PO Box 429
Addlestone
Surrey KT15 1DZ
Tel.: 01932 872560, 11 a.m. to 6 p.m. Monday to Friday

PREMSOC provides support for PMS self-help groups and individuals, runs
courses and publishes a newsletter. The staff answers general enquiries by
phone and post. Send an SAE for information and a publications list.

Royal College of Obstetricians and Gynaecologists (RCOG)
27 Sussex Place
Regent's Park
London NW1 4RG
Tel.: 020 7772 6200
Fax: 020 7723 0575
Website: www.rcog.urg.uk

This is the leading organization in the UK for healthcare professionals
working in women's health, with published guidelines on PMS.

Women's Nutritional Advisory Service
Natural Health Advisory Service
PO Box 117
Rottingdean
Brighton, East Sussex BN51 9BG
Tel.: 01273 609699
Fax: 01273 487576
Email: enquiries@naturalhealthas.com
Website: www.naturalhealthas.com

This service provides nutritional treatment for PMS. For a fee, your
symptoms, diet, medical history and lifestyle will be analysed and a
dietary treatment plan devised. There is access to counsellors by phone.

Index